A CARE CRISIS IN THE NORDIC WELFARE STATES?

Transforming Care

Series Editors: **Costanzo Ranci**,
Polytechnic University of Milan and
Tine Rostgaard, Stockholm University
and Roskilde University

Transforming Care provides a crucial platform for scholars
researching early childhood care, care for adults with
disabilities and long-term care for frail older people.
The series considers four dimensions of social care: the
institutional setting of care systems and policy; care
arrangements and practices; social and policy innovation
for care services and arrangements, and formal and
informal care work.

Forthcoming in the series:

Reablement in Long-term Care for Older People
By **Tine Rostgaard**

Find out more at
**policy.bristoluniversitypress.co.uk/
transforming-care**

A CARE CRISIS IN THE NORDIC WELFARE STATES?

Care Work, Gender Equality and Welfare State Sustainability

Edited by Lise Lotte Hansen,
Hanne Marlene Dahl and Laura Horn

First published in Great Britain in 2022 by

Policy Press, an imprint of
Bristol University Press
University of Bristol
1– 9 Old Park Hill
Bristol
BS2 8BB
UK
t: +44 (0)117 954 5940
e: bup- info@bristol.ac.uk

Details of international sales and distribution partners are available at:
policy.bristoluniversitypress.co.uk

© Bristol University Press 2022

British Library Cataloguing in Publication Data
A catalogue record for this book is available from the British Library

ISBN 978-1-4473-6134-3 hardcover
ISBN 978-1-4473-6136-7 ePub
ISBN 978-1-4473-6137-4 ePdf

Cover design by Robin Hawes
Image credit: istock/shuoshu

Printed and bound by CPI Group (UK) Ltd, Croydon, CR0 4YY

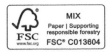

MIX
Paper | Supporting
responsible forestry
FSC® C013604

Contents

List of tables   vi
Notes on contributors   vii
Preface   ix

1   Introduction: A care crisis in the Nordic welfare states?   1
     Hanne Marlene Dahl and Lise Lotte Hansen

2   The 'care crisis': its scientific framing and silences   20
     Hanne Marlene Dahl

3   Fraser's care crisis theory meets the Nordic welfare societies   39
     Lise Lotte Hansen, Margunn Bjørnholt and Laura Horn

4   Crisis of care: a problem of economisation, of   60
     technologisation or of politics of care?
     Anne Kovalainen

5   Deteriorating working conditions in elder care: an invisible   80
     crisis of care?
     Anneli Stranz

6   Managerialism as a failing response to the care crisis   100
     *Hanna-Kaisa Hoppania, Antero Olakivi, Minna Zechner
     and Lena Näre*

7   'We are here for you': the care crisis and the (un)learning of   120
     good nursing
     Carsten Juul Jensen and Steen Baagøe Nielsen

8   Professionalisation of social pedagogues under managerial   139
     control: caring for children in a time of care crisis
     Steen Baagøe Nielsen

9   Raising quality in Norwegian early childhood centres: 158
     (re)producing the care crisis?
     Birgitte Ljunggren

10   Conclusion: Less caring and less gender-equal Nordic states   176
     Lise Lotte Hansen and Hanne Marlene Dahl

11   Postscript: A care crisis in the time of COVID-19   190
     Laura Horn, Carsten Juul Jensen and Birgitte Ljunggren

Index   200

List of tables

3.1   Core dimensions of Fraser's care crisis theory   44
3.2   Summary of care crisis dynamics in Nordic welfare societies   53
5.1   A two-dimensional conception of gender   83
8.1   Change of working conditions in ECECs: child–staff ratios   149
9.1   Overview of ECCs by number, competence measure scheme,   163
       ownership and number of informants

Notes on contributors

Margunn Bjørnholt is Professor in the Department of Sociology at the University of Bergen and Research Professor at Norwegian Centre for Violence and Traumatic Stress Studies (NKVTS), Oslo, Norway. Margunn is co-editor of *Men, Masculinities and Intimate Partner Violence* (with Gottzén et al, 2021).

Hanne Marlene Dahl holds a PhD in Political Science and is Professor in Social Science at Roskilde University, Denmark. Her main research is on the governance of care and its gendered aspects in the context of the Nordic, caring welfare states. She has recently published *Struggles in (Elderly) Care – A Feminist View* (2017), co-edited several books on care in a Nordic and European context and her latest publications have appeared in *International Journal of Care and Caring, Journal of Social Policy, Social Policy & Administration* and *Sociology of Health and Illness*.

Lise Lotte Hansen holds a PhD in Social Science. She is Associate Professor in Labour Market Studies and Head of the Center for Gender, Power and Diversity at Roskilde University, Denmark. She is the editor of *Køn, Magt & Mangfoldighed* (Frydenlund Academic, 2019). Lise Lotte also leads the Nordic Care Crisis Network.

Hanna-Kaisa Hoppania holds a PhD in Social Science and is interested in the politics of care. She currently works as Researcher at Age Institute, Helsinki, Finland, and from 2022 as Lecturer in Political Science and Sociology (Public and Social Policy) at National University of Ireland, Galway, Ireland. She has published in journals such as *Critical Social Policy, European Journal of Social Security,* and *Global Society.* She has also published with Routledge.

Laura Horn is Associate Professor in the Department of Social Science and Business at Roskilde University, Denmark. Her research is situated within critical political economy, focusing on capitalist restructuring in the European Union, social reproduction and economic and political imaginaries.

Carsten Juul Jensen is Lecturer at the Institute of Nursing and Health Sciences, University of Greenland, Denmark.

Anne Kovalainen holds a D.Sc(Econ.) in Economic Sociology and is Professor in Entrepreneurship at the University of Turku, Finland. She is a member of the Finnish Academy of Science and Letters, and the Finnish

Society of Sciences and Letters. Anne is co-editor of *Digital Work and the Platform Economy* (Routledge 2020), *Work and Labor in the Digital Age* (Emerald 2019) and co-author of *Gender and Innovation in the New Economy* (Palgrave 2017).

Birgitte Ljunggren is Associate Professor, Lecturer and Researcher at Queen Maud University College of Early Childhood Education, Trondheim, Norway. Her research focuses on leadership, management and governance in Early Childhood Education and Care (ECEC), as well as gender studies in ECEC. She is the co-editor of *Uadrettet barnehageledelse* (External leadership in ECEC, Universitetsforlaget 2021) and contributor to *Exploring Career Trajectories of Men in the Early Childhood Education and Care Workforce. Why They Leave and Why They Stay* (Routledge, 2021).

Lena Näre is Associate Professor of Sociology at the University of Helsinki, Finland. Lena is the editor-in-chief of *Nordic Journal of Migration Research* (Helsinki University Press) and associate editor of *Global Social Challenges Journal* (Bristol University Press).

Steen Baagøe Nielsen is Associate Professor in the Department of People and Technology at Roskilde University, Denmark.

Antero Olakivi is Postdoctoral Researcher at the University of Helsinki, Finland, in the Centre of Excellence in Research on Ageing and Care. His research focuses on care work and care work management, welfare state professionalism, and questions of identities, selfhood and interaction practices in work organisations.

Anneli Stranz is Senior Lecturer in Social Work at Stockholm University, Sweden, with a special research interest in governance and conditions of social care work in the Nordic welfare state. Her theoretical point of departure embrace gender justice, feminist welfare state theory and ethics of care.

Minna Zechner is Associate Professor in Social Work at the University of Lapland, Finland. Her research focuses mainly on elder care, recently focusing on capabilities in care, cash for care, new public governance, economisation and marketisation of care. Her works have been published in journals such as *Social Policy & Administration*, *International Journal of Care and Caring* and *Journal of Aging Studies*.

Preface

This book is the outcome of three years of in-depth discussions in the interdisciplinary Nordic Care Crisis Network (NCCN). The interest in the care crisis arose from a concern about what was happening to the Nordic welfare states. A wide range of problems had surfaced in our individual research, and there was a need to bring our respective expertise together to gain in-depth knowledge about various problems, to discuss their possible connections and useful ways of theorising a care crisis in the context of the Nordic welfare regime. We thank the network participants for insightful and important discussions.

We would also like to give thanks to the Nordic Council of Ministers, which has funded the network with means from the Gender Equality Fund. We would like to thank the Center for Nordic Information on Gender (NIKK), which administered the funding with great flexibility. Finally, we would like to express our gratitude to Professor Emerita Joan Tronto (University of Minnesota), who acted as a discussant to our work in progress papers and gave us valuable food for thought.

Lise Lotte Hansen, Hanne Marlene Dahl and Laura Horn

Introduction: A care crisis in the Nordic welfare states?

Hanne Marlene Dahl and Lise Lotte Hansen

Care, and being in need of care at various points of your life, is a condition of our existence. We can't live without giving and receiving care. You wouldn't be here reading this text without having been cared for as a baby. Being fed, bathed, nappies changed and having clean clothes put on. Care is embedded within practices in various institutional contexts, including the home, the hospital, the crèche and the nursing home. In these contexts most people are 'doing good' (Mol, 2007) in relation to those that are currently sick, disabled/challenged, children or fragile. Those that are doing less well need to receive help, support and coaching in a dialogic, ongoing, although possibly fragmented, process and adjust to the care provided. Throughout life we experience being dependent upon others to maintain our existence – or improve it. Care can be a burden, and care can create pleasant feelings of belonging, doing something together, doing good, and being seen as someone in need of care, or someone providing care. Care can be paid and unpaid, but regardless of this, it constitutes 'care work' as one of the founding mothers of Nordic care research, Kari Wærness, has argued (Wærness, 1982).

In this book we discuss the status of care work, and especially paid care work, in the Nordic welfare states in light of the neoliberal turn in welfare politics, and what this means for gender equality and the sustainability of the Nordic welfare state. When care work is commodified i.e. paid either in a market or by the state, it simultaneously becomes a public form of care work. Our focus is upon formalised care work, that is, care that is commodified (paid), regulated politically and 'performed' within the state or private institutions. By institutions we refer to conglomerations of practices in process (Bacchi and Rönnblom, 2014). The discussions in this book develop around the theoretical questions of what constitutes a care crisis, whether it can be expanded beyond its original application into a different context and rethought; a methodological question of its operationalisation (how to investigate it), and an empirical question about the justification of talking about a care crisis in the Nordic welfare states. Finally, we discuss the major areas of concern in terms of gender equality and elements of social sustainability in a situation of care crisis.

When care is talked about in politics today, it is typically seen as a financial burden (expenditure) or as a social investment, where investments in early childhood education and care are a way of investing in human capital and the conditions for successful lifelong learning in the competition between nations (OECD, 2001; EU Commission, 2011). In contrast – and as already mentioned – this book theorises care as a precondition for human life and human beings as interdependent (Tronto, 1991). Care is an analytical notion introduced by feminist sociologists (Wærness, 1982, 1987; Graham, 1983, 1991; Ungerson, 1983; Noddings, 1984) to describe a necessary, everyday occurrence of 'care work' that is marginalised, taken as given to be a freely-available good, or neglected. Today, care is increasingly a field of political attention and governance at various levels: local, national, internationally and supranationally (Milligan and Miles, 2010; Dahl, 2017). There is increasing political attention to care in its various forms; perhaps even a 'discursive explosion' with care being foregrounded in a situation of a global pandemic with COVID-19 (Chatzidakis et al, 2020: 890). However, even before the pandemic, there has been an increase in political will to govern care and an emerging – or sustained – politics of need interpretation (Fraser, 1989). Care becomes a field of political intervention, full of specific ideas of what constitutes good care (Dahl, 2017). Feminist economists would argue that care is the invisible heart of the society compared to the invisible hand of market economics (Folbre, 2001). In this sense, care is not an expenditure, but is at the core of the economy (Folbre, 2001; Bjørnholt and McKay, 2014) and its ultimate aim.

In the US and UK it has become commonplace to speak of a 'care crisis', especially in the media, with headlines such as: 'Jet-in carers fly from Benidorm to Britain amid "massive" care crisis' (*The Telegraph*, 2017). In this understanding of a care crisis, the issues are reduced to a recruitment crisis. In this book, however, we use and refer to a wider notion of a 'care crisis' – an analytical notion of a care crisis – which has been used for over two decades by care researchers (Phillips, 1994; Hochschild, 1995; Knijn and Kremer, 1997; Saraceno, 1997; Isaksen et al, 2008; Wrede et al, 2008; Tronto, 2013; Williams, 2018; The Care Collective, 2020). Originally, the notion referred to the decline of informal family-based care (based upon increasing participation of married/cohabiting women in paid labour) and the withdrawal of the welfare state. Recently the American philosopher Nancy Fraser has linked the care crisis to the relationship between productive and reproductive work and the predominance of a particular form of capitalism, namely financialised capitalism[1] (Fraser, 2016). While the literature speaks rather generally about a care crisis, or typically relates it to the Anglo-American context (Hochschild, 1995; Tronto, 2013), or a global care crisis (Isaksen et al, 2008), this book contextualises this discussion in another socio-political space. A space that is described as 'care friendly' (Vabø and Szebehely, 2012) and 'care work friendly' (Wrede et al, 2008). A space that is also defined as 'potentially women-friendly' states (Hernes, 1987), which in today's lingo translates into the supposedly more gender equal, Nordic welfare states of Denmark, Finland, Norway, Sweden and Iceland.

Why discuss a care crisis in the Nordic welfare states in which state responsibility for care services and the professionalisation of care work are already of major importance? The Nordic welfare model represents a 'passion for equality' (Hernes, 1987) that has been institutionalised as a political commitment to public-funded care services (Esping-Andersen, 1990) and to universalism. Universalism means that 'services are designed for all citizens, and in practice a large majority of citizens also use' them (Anttonen, 2002: 71). They are available to all when they need it and they are, generally, of good quality (Szebehely, 2003: 9). This universalism has enabled women to reconcile being mothers, daughters, workers and citizens, and increased the status of care work through care 'going public' and a state-supported – or state-engineered – professionalisation of care work (Dahl, 2010; Dahl and Rasmussen, 2012; Ulmanen, 2013). However, the Nordic welfare state model and the Nordic labour market model are exposed to major challenges following the turn to neoliberal politics and the financial crisis (Dahl, 2009, 2017; Poutanen and Kovalainen, 2014; Hansen, 2016). This has put pressure on care in various ways with the increasing focus upon individual responsibilities to self-care, welfare state retrenchment and/or austerity policies and the focus upon quality through 'documenting care'. Although neoliberalism is a transnational discourse, it travels into different institutional contexts. In this way the Nordic welfare states are latecomers to neoliberalism (Christensen and Lægreid, 2007), and reluctant ones; which makes them interesting cases to study how deeply neoliberalising effects – even care-friendly – states. Although we speak of the Nordic welfare states as one unit, it is an analytical construction (Kettunen, 2011) and these nations have also implemented different versions of neoliberalism. Research on elder care, for example, shows that different translations of neoliberalism have created a divide between the west (Norway and Denmark) and the east (Sweden and Finland). In the eastern part there has been a larger degree of retrenchment of elder care, more targeting of it and more outsourcing than in Norway and Denmark (Szebehely and Meagher, 2013). In this book, we are not ignoring the differences within the Nordic model discussed in the rich literature, but we are trying to take an outsider's and a bird's-eye view on its joint characteristics in terms of care in selected fields of interest.

The Nordic welfare states are often referred to as 'caring states' (Vabø and Szebehely, 2012). For feminists they are often considered to be feminist nirvanas, as care is not supposed to be solely the responsibility of women as unpaid work for significant others. Instead (most) care is seen as a state responsibility, tax-financed and provided by care professionals that enables women to combine paid and unpaid care work to be financially independent. The 'caring states' are a special case for discussing the relevance of the notion of a care crisis and can be characterised as a critical case. Bent Flyvbjerg defines a critical case as a case that permits logical deductions of this type: 'If this is (not) valid for this case, then it applies to all (no) cases' (Flyvbjerg, 2006: 230). The Nordic welfare states are a critical case as they are a *most unlikely case* for a care crisis to exist. The argument of this book is, therefore, that even in the best of circumstances in the supposedly feminist nirvana, there is a care crisis. That if a care crisis is valid for this case, then it applies to all cases. Readers will therefore agree with us in the following argument: if the concept of a 'care crisis' is relevant also for Nordic welfare regimes, then it is highly plausible that it is also highly relevant for other Western welfare regimes as well. The Nordic welfare states are a most unlikely case for a care crisis, so if a care crisis exists even here, the care crisis must be a more global phenomenon. In this book we move beyond the claim that there is a care crisis in the Nordic welfare states (although a smaller, and slightly different one, than in the original understandings of a care crisis) as we also argue that the concept of a 'care crisis' cannot simply be adopted from existing definitions but must be reworked (see Chapter 2 in this volume). Since knowledge is situated knowledge (Haraway, 1988) that is framed by and related to the context in question, we must reflect on how concepts travel to new contexts and whether they travel easily (Knapp, 2005; see also Chapter 2 in this volume). If key concepts are to travel, how can a good journey from one context to another be envisioned in a normative sense (Tronto, 2020)? Moreover, our book argues that care systematically relates to issues of gender equality and welfare state sustainability – and that the current developments challenge both elements. At the same time, the pressure on care, caring and care workers has led to significant social struggles nationally and globally (Dahl, 2017; Arruzza et al, 2018). This is where the Nordic context might make a difference.

Key concepts and rethinking the notion of a care crisis

In the following paragraphs we will define the key concepts of this book: *care*, *neoliberalism*, *care crisis* and *gender equality*. In doing so, we incorporate various analytical concepts under these umbrella terms that are used in the individual contributions to this book to discuss the Nordic care crisis issue.

As mentioned, care is one of the most important contributions of feminist theorising to social and political theory. However, it is contested in various competing understandings of what care is – and what it should be (Wærness, 1982; Ungerson, 1983; Noddings, 1984; Graham, 1991; Tronto, 1993; Bubeck, 1995; Kittay et al, 2005; Beasley and Bacchi, 2007;

Mol, 2007; Milligan and Wiles, 2010; Barnes, 2015; Dahl, 2017; de la Bellacasa, 2017; Urban and Ward, 2020). Whereas some view care as an attitude (Noddings, 1984), as a way of being in the world, others view care as a kind of rationality – different from other rationalities in the social world (Wærness, 1987). Still others view care as a circle of care (Bubeck, 1995); whereas Mol views care as a 'tinkering with care', with constant dialogue and negotiation of what defines the 'best' care (Mol, 2007). Increasingly, there is a focus upon the post-human, including the role of robots or computerised devices (the use of GPS in dementia care, robot seals and intelligent floors) and animals (such as dogs and cats) in care (Thygesen et al, 2013; de la Bellacasa, 2017; Hansen et al, 2018). Sometimes care is seen as consisting of practical and emotional support (Milligan and Wiles, 2010), whereas others stress practical, emotional *and* cognitive (knowledge-based) elements of care (Leira, 1994; Dahl, 2000). Some authors stress care as primarily one-directional – towards those being dependent upon others (Wærness, 1982). There is increasingly an understanding of care as involving multidirectional flows and connections (Milligan and Wiles, 2010). In this book, care is also seen as a resource that can be depleted (Buch, 2015); so instead of seeing care as a circle of care, it is nowadays seen as a circulation of care (Buch, 2015), with fragmentation and contingency (Thelen, 2015; Dahl, 2021) and even as an assemblage (Mol, 2007).

Inspired by Joan Tronto, among others, we view care as principally involving five schematically different aspects of care: caring about (seeing a need for care), taking care of (assuming some responsibility), care-giving (the direct meeting of needs for care), care-receiving (the response to care by the receiving person) and caring-with (Tronto, 1993, 2013). In this book we take a broad view of care as not just relational, between bodies or bodies and things, but as something that also involves the preconditions for human life, including cleaning: 'a species activity that includes everything we do to maintain, contain, and repair our "world" so that we can live in it as well as possible. That world includes our bodies, ourselves, and our environment, all of which we seek to interweave in a complex, life-sustaining web (Tronto and Fisher, 1990: 40). In this sense we try to avoid a dyadic view of care with only a giver and recipient of care. Identities are complex and contingent in the circulation of care. The current global pandemic has taught us that a concept of care that encompasses more than direct care for individuals can be meaningful (Bjørnholt, 2020).

Care is often used as a synonym for social reproduction, especially in the broad definition of care used above. In this book they are overlapping concepts that have different origins. Whereas the notion of 'care' is a feminist invention, 'reproduction' is an economic concept coined by the German social scientist Karl Marx. Social reproduction as a term refers to a central dynamic in capitalist society, in contrast to 'care' which is often not related to any economic system. In Fraser's words, 'reproduction' is 'an indispensable background condition for the possibility of capitalist production' (Fraser, 2014: 61). Social reproduction is about the processes, relations and activities which are necessary to maintain capitalist society, in particular the reproduction of labour power (Bhattacharya, 2017). Like in Tronto's broad concept of care, social reproduction activities include giving birth, bringing up children, teaching, caring for others, caring for oneself and for things, social relations and the earth – and it also includes 'producing and reproducing shared meanings, affective dispositions and horizons of value' (Fraser, 2014: 61). So despite differences in their genesis, the two concepts are applied as synonyms in this book.

Neoliberalism and neoliberalising are widely used terms but are not often defined. They are used interchangeably with the notion of New Public Management (NPM), although epistemologically and theoretically they have different origins (Dahl, 2012). Both are transnational, complex and dynamic discourses. Whereas neoliberalism takes a broad view of the state, and its relationship with and effects upon the economy and civil society, NPM directs our attention to what is happening within the state in terms of reforms. Neoliberalism forms a political-economic governance that extends the logic of the market, individualisation and responsibility into all areas of social life. It redefines the state as subservient to the economy and produces calculating subjects instead of rule-abiding ones (Larner, 2000; Brown, 2003). NPM stressing the need for the marketisation of services and the use of management techniques by the state that stress the importance of professional leadership, self-engineering and self-motivation (Hood, 1991; Andersen, 2001; Sahlin-Andersson, 2002; Dahl, 2011). Often the buzzwords have been 'better and cheaper' services when arguing in favour of the implementation of NPM. There is substantial literature on NPM in the Nordic welfare states which, compared to its Anglo-American counterparts, show that the Nordic welfare states are both latecomers to NPM and apply 'NPM-light' (Christensen and Lægreid, 2007; Sahlin-Andersson, 2002; Greve, 2003; Dahl, 2009). The emphasis on equality within the Nordic welfare states has profound implications for the conversion of NPM as it translates into an expansion in the regulation of care and its standardisation to ensure a control of service provision (Dahl, 2011; Dahl and Rasmussen, 2012).[2] Feminist scholars have identified negative effects of neoliberalism and NPM on care. Tronto, for example, has argued that neoliberalism becomes the antithesis of a caring society and caring human beings (Tronto, 2017). Neoliberalising, over time, co-opts new terms, for example 'empowerment', and rearticulates old ones (Dahl, 2009; Newman and Tonkens, 2011). Neoliberalising threatens care by changing the logics – and inner workings – of care provided by care professionals, their identities, responsibilities and ideals of good care by creating a 'thin', stoic version of care (Dahl, 2012). For some, this has led to discussions of a care squeeze and a care crisis.

As previously mentioned, in the Anglo-American countries there is a dominant media narrative of a health care crisis, and also a scientific narrative of a care crisis in the UK and US (Phillips, 1994; Hochschild, 1995; Haraham, 2011; *The Lancet*, 2014; Roberts, 2018; Dowling, 2021). This is not the case in the Nordic countries, where there has been no public debate that mentions a 'care crisis'. Except in Finland where politicians now refer to a 'national care crisis' (see Chapter 6 in this volume). The question then becomes how to define a care crisis and its characteristics. In the scientific literature, there are two competing frameworks of a care crisis: Arlie R. Hochschild's (Hochschild, 1995; Isaksen et al, 2008) and Nancy Fraser's (2016; Arruzza et al, 2018). Hochschild views a care crisis as consisting of a national crisis and a global one. The national crisis (with a reference to the US) consists of increasing needs for care with declining resources for giving care. The latter relates to the increasing number of dual-earner families, single-parent families and welfare state retrenchment, and the care crisis refers to insufficient resources, both financially and of (wo)manpower. There are insufficient funds and hands allocated to care. This care crisis in the Global North gives impetus to global and regional migration where care workers and professional carers from the Global South travel and stay in the Global North, working in families and institutions providing care. This care drain results in declining commons in the communities left behind by, the primarily female, migrants; thereby creating a global care crisis (Isaksen et al, 2008). In contrast, Fraser considers the care crisis the result of an inherent contradiction in capitalism exacerbated by financialised capitalism, with an increasing extraction and a neoliberal state (Fraser, 2016). Fraser redefines the main contradiction in capitalism as one between production and social reproduction, where social reproduction is seriously threatened. Whereas Hochschild primarily relates the care crisis to changes in civil society and the state, Fraser directs our attention to the economy and, to a lesser extent, the state and different state strategies. What is missing is an analysis of how care within the state – and regulated by the state – changes with neoliberalism, and what kind of care is the result of neoliberal care as managerialised care, with less autonomy for those actually doing the care. Neoliberal care results in 'thin' care due to an increasing amount of bureaucracy, documentation and standardising care with less time for hands-on care (Dahl, 2012). At the same time, neoliberal care offloads care to families and significant others and articulates a particular ideal of care as the self-responsible, active and self-caring person. Neoliberal care tries to capitalise on the resources of communities with state and non-governmental organisations (NGOs), focusing upon engineering voluntariness (Regeringen, 2010; Muehlenbach, 2012).

Building on Fraser (2016), Hochschild (1995) and Phillips (1994) we want to develop a more contextualised notion of a care crisis that fits the Nordic welfare states. Hochschild introduces in her early work different kinds of ideal-typical forms of care, where the notions of 'cold-modern' and 'postmodern care' (Hochschild, 1995) are relevant in the contemporary Nordic context. The cold-modern ideal of care refers to a situation where care is institutionalised, pressing for maximum hours and institutional control. Care in a cold-modern ideal is seen as 'practical, efficient and rational' (Hochschild, 1995: 341). In contrast, the postmodern ideal of care describes a situation with a dual-breadwinner model where major parts of care are institutionalised, but where women still perform more care than men in relation to formalised care work and care in families, and in extended models of kinship. Women seem to be 'doing it all', although masculinity is on the move. In Hochschild's view, postmodern care becomes a 'stoic' form of care with reduced expectations and obligations to care. Care – and care needs – are rewritten. Fraser directs our attention to the inherent contradiction and depletion of resources for care in capitalism, its various 'stages' and state strategies. Phillips turns our attention to the professional carers in industries of caring, concerning their conditions for providing good care. In this sense, we define a care crisis as characterised by inadequate resources for care and the absence of 'good-enough' care – the latter a term introduced by sociologist Fiona Williams(1999).[3] The term 'inadequate resources' refers to insufficient economic resources to meet the wishes for, and needs of, care. From surveys conducted in two major Finnish cities, in 2010 and 2015, Kröger et al showed that there is an inadequate coverage of care needs among the elderly, especially among poor, sick elderly that live alone (Kröger et al, 2019). Cracks begin to show in the façade of care within the Nordic welfare states.

The Nordic welfare states have been called 'potentially women-friendly' (Hernes, 1987). However, if they are 'women-friendly' at all *and* if a 'women-friendly' approach is the best way to discuss gender power relations and politics have been widely questioned (Holst, 2006; Dahl, 2010). The critique points at too much focus on agency and on paid labour, and too little focus on differences between women; although Helga Hernes (1987) mentioned differences among women as a major challenge to gender equality. The emphasis on equality in labour market participation has contributed to the reproduction of a male norm regarding labour (Holst, 2006). Simultaneously, there is growing inequality between women depending on generation, ethnicity and class (Borchorst and Siim, 2008); and a labour market horizontally and vertically segregated according to gender (Christensen and Siim, 2001). In Nordic gender research, 'women-friendliness' has been replaced by the concept of gender equality, emphasising the relationality of gendered power *and* of intersecting inequality dynamics. This is what we will call a *'gender equality +'* perspective, which pays attention to gendered power relations that include intersectional perspectives on gender equality, such as class and ethnicity, as mentioned previously, which include other axes of inequalities or markers of difference.

Gender equality is essentially contested both scientifically and politically. It is a floating signifier. As a policy goal, gender equality depends on the objectives, strategies and tools used. Gender equality policies are context-dependent and are influenced by political discourses, which from a care crisis point of view makes neoliberal gender equality policies part of the problem (Fraser, 2016; Bhattacharya et al, 2018). In addition, gender equality policies are not only a solution to specific inequalities, but they also constitute specific problem representations. Gender equality policies constitute gender equality as a specific problem, silencing other representations (Bacchi, 1999, 2009). Implicit in the term 'gender equality' is a balance–perspective: that women and men should be equal. In a broader understanding, we can talk about an equal distribution of power, resources and dignity (Borchorst and Dahlerup, 2003). The new feminist movements, however, call for more radical changes that go beyond gender equality, and just like the feminism of the 1960s and 1970s, they speak about liberation as including respect for care work and for care-givers (Arruzza et al, 2018). This tension between equality and liberation is fundamental to gender equality policies as well as the continuous contestation of what equality is. Gender equality is more than just the absence of discrimination and is instead about gendered justice understood as an issue of distribution, recognition and representation (Fraser, 2008). Although feminists have discussed gender equality for centuries (Wollstonecraft, 1792; Jonasdottir, 1991; Scott, 2009), little has been published regarding equality in relation to care, care work and its gendered characteristics. However, these topics have been discussed by two theorists: Fraser introduced the notion of the 'universal carer' (Fraser, 1997) and Hochschild the notion of the 'warm modern model' (Hochschild, 1995). Both ideals stress the equal distribution of care between men and women (degendering care), recognition of care as important, vital work ('warm') and the role of public (read: state) institutions in provision of care. Only with access to, and availability of, public care, can women combine paid work, daughterhood and motherhood. The state can also – as seen in the Nordic countries – contribute to some recognition of care as paid, important work (Dahl, 2010).

Focus and limits of this book

As there is no research on a care crisis in the Nordic welfare states, except an edited book from 2008 (Wrede et al, 2008), this book is exploratory – showing results from four countries and selected fields: pre-school care, elderly in need of care (the oldest old) and care of the sick in hospitals. These fields are crucial to gender equality, enabling women to be daughters/

daughters–in–law and mothers, while earning their own living in the paid labour market. These three fields are characterised by mostly being composed of women working as care professionals, and through the ongoing struggle about the recognition of care.

This book is neither comparative, nor the outcome of a joint research project with a common theoretical framework. Instead it is the result of research carried out by individual researchers that recognise the need for specific, in–depth studies. In our research, we discovered how difficult it was to use existing elder care data to make scientific statements about the existence of a care crisis. This realisation was in terms of a changing number of elderly, changing needs and changing policy measures, such as 'everyday rehabilitation' ('re–ablement') and how these trends relate to the number of employed professionals and the resources available.

The presence of case material from four of the Nordic countries allows readers to develop a richer understanding of the different ways that these states are now thinking about matters of care in neoliberal times. Studying care in particular contexts is in line with what care researchers within Science Technology Studies, anthropology, sociology and geography have argued: that care needs to be studied within various practices to 'get a grip of what's going on'. By doing so, these researchers highlight the complexity, heterogeneity and ambivalence of care, and of 'doing good' (Mol, 2007; Mol et al, 2010; Moser and Pols, 2010; Buch, 2015).

The following chapters include different views of what constitutes a care crisis, its causes and of how to use theories of care crisis in a Nordic context; most contributions refer to Fraser's notion of a care crisis. 'Women–friendly' is traditionally used as a reference point for feminist analyses, but in this book various forms of feminist perspectives are applied that seek to be aware of – and reflect upon – the intersections of gender, ethnicity and class. Therefore, chapters apply a gender perspective and – to various extents – consider the lived effects of various policies (Bacchi, 2009). The feminist analyses in this book are from the perspective of a 'critical insider', where feminists deconstruct the myth of a women–friendly welfare state and point to cracks in the façade of the feminist nirvana. These are critical analyses of states that are usually understood as caring. It is a theoretical lens with which to view the global discussion of the quality of care. We have not applied intersectionality systematically in this exploratory work as this would require more in–depth studies.

Contributions to the field

This book contributes to the emerging, scientific literature on a care crisis in an unusual context; that of the so–called 'care-friendly' welfare states in Northern Europe. It does so through theoretical and exploratory methodological discussions, as well as providing empirical knowledge about the current state of public care in different states and settings, such as kindergartens, hospitals and elder care, characterised by neoliberalising. The book starts with theoretical discussions in Chapters 2 and 3 and ends in investigations of specific cases in different nations and forms of care.

In Chapter 2, Hanne Marlene Dahl digs into the scientific archives and gives us historical knowledge of the framing of the care crisis theoretically. The 'care crisis' is a concept that was 'born in the USA' in a liberal welfare regime with a rampant neoliberalising more than two decades ago. This framing of the care crisis doesn't travel easily to other regimes such as the social-democratic welfare regimes, where it silences important aspects of care such as professional care and issues of good care. Dahl argues that researchers need to reflect upon their 'scientific backpack', their framing of the care crisis and rethink the concept to fit the context, as well as recover lost insights from the early theorising of the care crisis.

Chapter 3 continues the theoretical discussion but takes its point of departure from Nancy Fraser's understanding of a care crisis. The authors, Lise Lotte Hansen, Margunn Bjørnholt and Laura Horn, are 'thinking with' Nancy Fraser and her theorising of the care crisis, and they argue that it can be applied to the Nordic context and operationalised into five dimensions – in effect making a restatement of her theorising. Furthermore, they argue empirically that there is a care crisis, although different and less severe in the Nordic countries than elsewhere. They take a specific look at financialised capitalism at work in care, devaluation of care work in families and elements of resistance to neoliberalising and financialisation in the labour market.

In Chapter 4, Anne Kovalainen identifies three disconnected scientific fields and discourses about care ethics, economy (marketisation/outsourcing) and technologies in care. In the context of the Nordic welfare states, she argues that we need a deeper understanding of capitalism and neoliberalism in order to understand the specific, historical context – and why a technological fix has become so prevalent in political discourses on care, especially in health and elder care.

Chapter 5 is written by Anneli Stranz. Her point of departure is working conditions for care professionals in elder care. Based upon a major survey in collaboration with others and applying Fraser's original two-dimensional theorising on justice (redistribution and recognition), she argues that there is an invisible crisis in elder care. This is based upon the replies of the professional carers stressing mental, emotional and bodily fatigue and understaffing – a working life that can feed into higher turnover – and consequently, of increasing recruitment problems. Stranz ends her contribution with a cautious, optimistic note quoting the Swedish prime minister in favour of allocating more resources to elder care, as a possible response to the high death rates in Swedish nursing homes related to COVID-19.

In Chapter 6, Hanna-Kaisa Hoppania, Antero Olakivi, Minna Zechner and Lena Näre continue the discussion on elder care, this time in Finland, and take a deeper look at the prevailing neoliberal discourses and what this does to elder care. In Finland, policy-makers have begun to talk about a 'national care crisis' in elder care, making it a topic of political discussion – and so no longer exclusively discussed in academic texts. The authors identify an endemic crisis in elder care based upon neoliberalism and its focus upon good leadership in the discourse of managerialism. They argue that we need to direct our attention to the governance of care itself as it becomes part of the problem; that the solution (better management) becomes part of the problem (bad elder care) in a vicious circle. In this way, managerialism directs our attention away from the main drivers of a care crisis: understaffing and underfinancing.

In Chapter 7, we turn to health care and hospitals in the Danish context. Carsten Juul Jensen and Steen Baagøe Nielsen report upon the way neoliberalising stresses efficiency and consumer-oriented services in hospitals, and how this is experienced by newly qualified nurses based upon institutional ethnographic research. Jensen and Baagøe Nielsen identify the struggle between philosophies of caring (ethics of care) and their everyday lives, discussing the guilt, shame and emotional breakdowns of nurses. These young nurses have to unlearn the ideals of care taught in nursing schools to adapt to the harsh realities of working life in hospitals, and the authors identify a gender difference in their work practices, that may or may not be representative of gender differences generally within nursing. The authors discuss the notions of a 'care crisis' in relation to a less serious situation, that of a 'care squeeze'.

Chapter 8 is written by Steen Baagøe Nielsen. He explores professionalisation in a context of Danish kindergartens encountering NPM with its bureaucratic measurement and evidence-based 'toolbox' programmes. Listening to the voices of seven newly graduated pedagogues that work in kindergartens, Baagøe Nielsen argues that they experience major difficulties maintaining their professional identity attained at university colleges. They feel overwhelmed and helpless as they encounter the double pressure from cuts (underfunding) and a reorientation of their daily work towards that which can be monitored and valued. This form of professionalisation becomes a double-edged sword that feeds into a Nordic care crisis by rationalising and reorganising public care.

In Chapter 9, Birgitte Ljunggren takes us to from Danish to Norwegian kindergartens. Here, she directs our attention to a core element of the social investment paradigm, that of continuously raising the competences of the staff. Staff in the Nordic context may be either professionally educated carers ('pedagogues') or unskilled assistants. Based upon seven cases and interviews with leaders, pedagogical leaders, professional carers and unskilled assistants,

Ljunggren argues that there is a cross pressure between the child-centred logic of the kindergarten and competence-raising projects. Competence schemes of the government become a potential time thief, removing the staff from the children. The daily rhythm of the kindergartens is maintained but with different tempos where time strategies are applied to make ends meet; multitasking and the postponing of tasks becomes more frequent.

Lise Lotte Hansen and Hanne Marlene Dahl conclude the book in Chapter 10. They develop cross-cutting issues and discuss the consequences of a care crisis for gender equality and welfare state sustainability. Hansen and Dahl revisit the Nordic welfare state as a critical case arguing that there are both vicious and virtuous elements as well as lessons to be learned going beyond the Nordic care regimes. Finally, they outline some avenues for future research.

This book was almost finished when COVID-19 hit the world. We decided to add a postscript, and Laura Horn, Carsten Juul Jensen and Birgitte Ljunggren provide vignettes on the current situation of COVID-19. Through poems and letters they reflect on their personal experiences in the midst of a global pandemic, bringing to the fore memories, fears, frustrations and delights; a truly ambiguous situation in relation to different forms of care.

Notes

[1] Financialised capitalism is a form of capitalism where profits derive from interests, rents and dividends.

[2] Although Jakob Torfing and Peter Triantafillou have different interpretations of NPM and believe that standardisation is inherent in NPM (Torfing and Triantafillou, 2017).

[3] 'Good-enough' care refers to care that relate to values such as bodily integrity and voice of those at the receiving end.

References

Andersen, N.Å. (2001) *Kærlighed og omstilling – Italesættelsen af den offentligt ansatte*, Copenhagen: Nyt fra samfundsvidenskaberne.

Anttonen, A. (2002) 'Universalism and social policy: A Nordic-feminist revaluation', *NORA*, 10(2): 71–80.

Arruzza, C., Bhattacharya, T. and Fraser, N. (2018) 'Notes for a feminist manifesto', *New Left Review*, 114: 113–134.

Bacchi, C. (1999) *Women, Policy and Politics: The Construction of Policy Problems*, London: SAGE.

Bacchi, C. (2009) *What's the Problem Represented to Be?* French Forests: Pearson.

Bacchi, C. and Rönnblom, M. (2014) 'Feminist discursive institutionalism: A post-structuralist alternative, *NORA*, 22(3): 170–186.

Barnes, M. (2015) 'Beyond the dyad: Exploring the multidimensionality of care' in M. Barnes and T. Brannelly (eds) *Ethics of Care: Critical Advances in International Perspective*, Bristol: Policy Press, pp 31–44.

Beasley, C. and Bacchi, C. (2007) 'Envisaging a new politics for an ethical future: Beyond trust, care and generosity – towards an ethic of "social flesh"', *Feminist Theory*, 8(3): 279–298.

Bhattacharya, T. (2017) 'Introduction: Mapping social reproduction theory' in T. Bhattacharya (ed) *Social Reproduction Theory: Remapping Class, Recentering Oppression*, London: Pluto Press, pp 1–20.

Bjørnholt, M. (2020) 'Care, work and the creation of value in the pandemic', *Cambio*, OpenLab on Covid-19. DOI: 10.13128/cambio-8995

Bjørnholt, M. and McKay, A. (eds) (2014) *Counting on Marilyn Waring: New Advances in Feminist Economics*, Bradford: Demeter Press.

Borchorst, A. and Dahlerup, D. (2003) *Ligestillingspolitik som diskurs og praksis*, Frederiksberg: Samfundslitteratur.

Borchorst, A. and Siim, B. (2008) 'Women friendly policies and state feminism', *Feminist Theory*, 9(2): 207–224.

Brown, W. (2003) 'Neo–liberalism and the end of liberal democracy', *Theory and Event*, 7(1). Available from: http://muse.jhu.edu/journals/theory_and_event/v007/7.1brown.html [accessed 26 June 2021].

Bubeck, D. (1995) *Care, Gender and Justice*, Oxford: Clarendon Press.

Buch, E.D. (2015) 'Anthropology of aging and care', *Annual Review of Anthropology*, 44: 277–293.

The Care Collective (2020) *The Care Manifesto*, London: Verso.

Chatziadis, A., Hakim, J., Littler, J., Rottenberg, C. and Segal, L. (2020) 'From care washing to radical care: The discursive explosion of care during Covid-19', *Feminist Media Studies*, 20(6): 889–895.

Christensen, T. and Lægreid, P. (2007) 'Theoretical approach and research questions' in T. Christensen and P. Lægreid (eds) *Transcending New Public Management: The Transformation of Public Sector Reform*, Aldershot: Ashgate, pp 1–16.

Christensen, A.-D. and Siim, B. (2001) 'Den danske kønspolitiske model i et komparativt perspektiv' in A.-D. Christensen and B. Siim (eds) *Køn, demokrati og modernitet. Mod nye politiske horisonter*, København: Hans Reitzels Forlag, pp 39–60.

Dahl, H.M. (2000) 'A perceptive and reflective state?', *European Journal of Women's Studies*, 7(4): 475–494.

Dahl, H.M. (2009) 'New public management, care and struggles about recognition', *Critical Social Policy*, 29(4): 634–654.

Dahl, H.M. (2010) 'An old map of state feminism and an insufficient recognition of care', *NORA*, 18(3): 152–166.

Dahl, H.M. (2011) 'Who can be against quality? A new story about home-based care: NPM and governmentality', in C. Ceci, K. Björnsdottir and M.E. Purkis (eds) *Perspectives on Care at Home for Older People*, London: Routledge, pp 139–157.

Dahl, H.M. (2012) 'Neo-liberalism meets the Nordic welfare states: Gaps and silences', *NORA*, 20(4): 283–288.

Dahl, H.M. (2017) *Struggles in (Elderly) Care: A Feminist View*, London: Palgrave Macmillan.

Dahl, H.M. (2021) 'Strangers in care: Using fiction to re-theorize care for the oldest old', *International Journal of Care and Caring*, e-pub ahead of print. DOI: https://doi.org/10.1332/239788221X16099490162894

Dahl, H.M. and Rasmussen, B. (2012) 'Paradoxes in elder care: The Nordic model' in A. Kamp and H. Hvid (eds) *Elder care in Transition: Management, Meaning and Identity at Work. A Scandinavian Perspective*, Copenhagen: Copenhagen Business School Press, pp 29–49.

de la Bellacasa, M.P. (2017) *Matters of Care: Speculative Ethics in More Than Human Worlds*, Minneapolis: Minnesota University Press.

Dowling, E. (2021) *The Care Crisis: What Caused It and How Can We End It?* London: Verso.

Esping-Andersen, G. (1990) *Three Worlds of Welfare Capitalism*, Oxford: Polity Press.

EU Commission (2011) *Early Childhood Education and Care: Providing All Our Children with the Best Start for the World of Tomorrow*, Communication from the Commission 17.2. COM 66, Available from: https://eur-lex.europa.eu/LexUriServ/LexUriServ.do?uri=COM:2011:0066:FIN:EN:PDF [accessed 23 November 2020].

Fisher, B. and Tronto, J. (1990) 'Toward a feminist theory of caring' in E. Abel and M.K. Nelson (eds) *Circles of Care: Work and Identity in Women's Lives*, Albany: SUNY Press, pp 35–62.

Flyvbjerg, B. (2006) 'Five misunderstandings about case study research', *Qualitative Inquiry*, 12(2): 219–245.

Folbre, N. (2001) *The Invisible Heart: Economics and Family Values*, New York: New Press.

Fraser, N. (1989) 'Talking about needs: Interpretive contests as political conflicts in welfare state societies', *Ethics*, 99(2): 291–313.

Fraser, N. (1997) *Justice Interruptus*, New York and London: Routledge.

Fraser, N. (2008) *Scales of Justice: Reimagining Political Space in a Globalizing World*, New York: Columbia University Press.

Fraser, N. (2009) 'Feminism, capitalism and the cunning of history', *New Left Review*, 56: 99.

Fraser, N. (2014) 'Behind Marx's hidden abode: For an expanded conception of capitalism', *New Left Review*, 86 (March/April): 55–72.

Fraser, N. (2016) 'Contradictions of capital and care', *New Left Review* 100(July/August): 99.

Graham, H. (1983) 'Caring: A labour of love' in J. Finch and D. Groves (eds) *A Labour of Love: Women, Work and Caring*, London: RKP, pp 13–30.

Graham, H. (1991) 'The concept of caring in feminist research', *Sociology*, 25(1): 507–515.

Greve, C. (2003) *Offentlig ledelse: Teorier og temaer i et politologisk perspektiv*, Copenhagen: Jurist- og Økonomforbundets Forlag.

Hansen, L.L. (2016) 'Er den danske model kvindevenlig? Den Danske Arbejdsmarkedsmodel set fra en udefra-indefra position' in A. Ilsøe and T.P. Larsen (eds) *Den Danske Model set udefra*, Copenhagen: Jurist- og Økonomforbundets Forlag, pp 385–408.

Hansen, A.M., Kamp, A. and Grosen, S.L. (2018) 'Velfærdsteknologi mellem ansvar og distance', *Arbejdsliv*, 20(3): 24–40.

Haraham, M.F. (2011) 'A critical look at the looming long-term-care workforce crisis', *Generations: Journal of the American Society on Ageing*, 34(4): 20–26.

Haraway, D. (1988) 'Situated knowledges: The science question in feminism and the privilege of perspective', *Feminist Studies*, 14(3): 575–599.

Hernes, H. (1987) *Welfare State and Woman Power: Essays in State Feminism*, Oslo: Universitetsforlaget.

Hochschild, A.R. (1995) 'The culture of politics: Traditional, postmodern, cold-modern and warm-modern ideals of care', *Social Politics*, 2(3): 331–346.

Holst, C. (2006) 'Statsfeminismen og nasjonalstaten', *Kvinder, Køn & Forskning*, 15(4): 5–16.

Hood, C. (1991) 'A public management for all seasons?', *Public Administration*, 69(1): 3–19.

Isaksen, L.W., Devi, U.S. and Hochschild, A.R. (2008) 'Global care crisis: A problem of capital, care chain, or commons?', *American Behavioral Scientist*, 52(3): 405–425.

Jonasdottir, A.G. (1991) *Love Power and Political Interests*, Örebro: Örebro Studies.

Kettunen, P. (2011) 'The transational construction of national challenges' in P. Kettunen and K. Petersen (eds) *Beyond Welfare State Models*, Cheltenham: Edward Elgar, pp 16–40.

Kittay, E., Jennings, B. and Wasunna, A. (2005) 'Dependency, difference and the global ethic of longterm care', *The Journal of Political Philosophy*, 13(4): 443–469.

Knapp, G. (2005) 'Race, class, gender: Reclaiming baggage in fast travelling theories', *European Journal of Women's Studies*, 12(3): 249–265.

Knijn, T. and Kremer, M. (1997) 'Gender and the caring dimension of the welfare states: Towards inclusive citizenship', *Social Politics*, 4(3): 328–361.

Kröger, T., Puthenparabil, J.M. and Aerschot, L. (2019) 'Care poverty: Unmet care needs in a Nordic welfare state', *International Journal of Care and Caring*, 3(4): 485–500.

The Lancet (2014) 'Editorial: Global elder care in crisis', *The Lancet*, 383(9921): 927.

Larner, W. (2000) 'Neo-liberalism: Policy, ideology and governmentality', *Studies in Political Economy*, 63(3): 5–26.

Leira, A. (1994) 'The concept of caring: Loving, thinking, and doing', *Social Service Review*, 68(2): 185–201.

Milligan, C. and Miles, J. (2010) 'Landscapes of care', *Progress in Human Geography*, 34(1): 736–754.

Mol, A. (2007) *The Logic of Care: Health and the Problem of Patient Choice*, London: Routledge.

Mol, A., Moser, I. and Pols, J. (2010) 'Care: Putting practice into theory' in A. Mol, I. Moser and J. Pols (eds) *Care in Practice: On Tinkering in Clinics, Homes and Farms*, Bielefeld: Transcript Verlag, pp 7–25.

Muehlenbach, A. (2012) *The Moral Neoliberal: Welfare and Citizenship in Italy*, Chicago: Chicago University Press.

Newman, J. and Tonkens, E. (2011) 'Introduction' in J. Newman and E. Tonkens (eds) *Participation, Responsibility and Choice: Summoning the Active Citizen in Western European Welfare States*, Amsterdam: Amsterdam University Press, pp 9–28.

Noddings, N. (1984) *Caring: A Feminine Approach to Ethics and Moral Education*, Berkeley: University of California Press.

OECD (2001) *Starting Strong: Early Childhood Education and Care*, Paris: OECD.

Phillips, S.S. (1994) 'Introduction' in S.S. Phillips and P. Benner (eds) *The Crisis of Care: Affirming and Restoring Care Practices in Helping Professions*, Washington, DC: Georgetown University Press, pp 1–15.

Poutanen, S. and Kovalainen, A. (2014) 'What is new in the "new economy"? Care as critical nexus challenging rigid conceptualizations' in J. Gruchlich and B. Riegraf (eds) *Transnational Spaces and Gender*, Münster: Westfälisches Dampfboot, pp 176–192.

Regeringen (2010) *National civilsamfundsstrategi*, Copenhagen: Socialministeriet. Available from: https://www.ft.dk/samling/20101/almdel/sou/bilag/17/900000.pdf [accessed 23 November 2020].

Roberts, C. (2018) 'A crisis of care or a crisis of work', *IPPR Progressive Review*, 25(3): 302–311.

Sahlin-Andersson, K. (2002) 'National, international and transnational constructions of new public management' in T. Christensen and P. Lægreid (eds) *New Public Management: The Transformation of Ideas and Practice*, Aldershot: Ashgate, pp 43–73.

Saraceno, C. (1997) *Family, Market and Community*, Paris: OECD.

Scott, J.W. (2009) *Only Paradoxes to Offer: French Feminism and the Rights of Man*, Cambridge, MA: Harvard University Press.

Szebehely, M. (2003) 'Den nordiske hemtjänsten – bakgrund och omfatning' in M. Szebehely (ed) *Hemhjälp i Norden – illustrationer og reflektioner*, Lund: Studentlitteratur, pp 23–61.

Szebehely, M. and Meagher, G. (2013) 'Four Nordic countries: Four responses to the international trend of marketization' in G. Meagher and M. Szebehely (eds) *Marketization in Nordic Elder care*, Stockholm: Department of Social Work, pp 241–283.

The Telegraph (2017) 'Jet-in carers fly from Benidorm to Britain amid "massive" care crisis', 1 January.

Thelen, T. (2015) 'Care as a social organization: Creating, maintaining and dissolving significant relation', *Anthropological Theory*, 15(4): 497–515.

Torfing, J. and Triantafillou, P. (2017) 'Introduktion: New public governance på dansk' in J. Torfing and P. Triantafillou (eds) *New Public Management på dansk*, Copenhagen: Akademisk forlag, pp 7–39.

Tronto, J. (1993) *Moral Boundaries: A Political Argument for an Ethic of Care*, New York: Routledge.

Tronto, J. (2013) *Caring Democracy: Markets, Equality, and Justice*, New York: Routledge.

Tronto, J. (2017) 'There is an alternative: *Hominens Curans* and the limits of neo-liberalism', *International Journal of Care and Caring*, 1(1): 27–43.

Tronto, J. (2020) 'Caring democracy: How should concepts travel?' in P. Urban and L. Ward (eds) *Care Ethics, Democratic Citizenship and the State*, Cham: Palgrave Macmillan, pp 181–197.

Ulmanen, P. (2013) 'Working daughters: A blind spot in Swedish elder care policy', *Social Politics*, 20(1): 65–87.

Ungerson, C. (1983) 'Women and caring: Skills, tasks, and taboos' in E. Garmanikow, D.H.J. Morgan, J. Purvis and D. Taylorson (eds) *The Public and the Private*, London: Heinemann, pp 62–77.

Urban, P. and Ward, L. (2020) 'Introduction' in P. Urban and L. Ward (eds) *Care Ethics, Democratic Citizenship and the State*, Cham: Palgrave Macmillan, pp 1–27.

Vabø, M. and Szebehely, M. (2012) 'A caring state for all older people?' in A. Anttonen, L. Häikö and K. Stefasson (eds) *Welfare State, Universalism and Diversity*, Cheltenham: Edward Elgar, pp 212–243.

Wærness, K. (1982) *Kvinneperspektiver på Socialpolitikken*, Oslo: Universitetsforlaget.

Wærness, K. (1987) 'On the rationality of caring' in A. Sassoon (ed) *Women and the State*, London: Hutchinson, pp 207–234.

Willliams, F. (1999) 'Good enough principles for welfare', *Journal of Social Policy*, 28(4): 667–687.

Williams, F. (2018) 'Care: Intersections of scales, inequalities and crises', *Current Sociology*, 66(4): 547–561.

Wollstonecraft, M. (1792) *A Vindication of the Rights of Woman*, Cambridge: Cambridge University Press.

Wrede, S., Henriksson, L., Høst, H., Johansson, S. and Dybbroe, B. (2008) 'Introduction: Care work and the competing rationalities of public policy' in S. Wrede, L. Henriksson, H. Høst, S. Johansson and B. Dybbroe (eds) *Care Work in Crisis: Reclaiming the Nordic Ethos of Care*, Lund: Studentlitteratur, pp 15–37.

2

The 'care crisis': its scientific framing and silences

Hanne Marlene Dahl

Introduction

The Nordic welfare regimes are often referred to as 'caring states' (Vabø and Szebehely, 2012), care-work-friendly (Wrede et al, 2008), social–democratic welfare regimes characterised by universalism (Esping-Andersen, 1990) and as potentially women-friendly welfare states (Hernes, 1987). However, major changes have taken place within these welfare regimes prompted by policies promoting neoliberalism and austerity. Neoliberalising[1] has involved a wave of change with marketisation (contracting out) of elder care, self-responsibilising the elderly with concepts of 'self-care' and 're-ablement' as well as the increasing amount of documentation, performance measurement and quality control in institutions providing care (Clarke and Newman, 1997; Meagher and Szebehely, 2013; Dahl et al, 2015; Dahl, 2017). Simultaneously, there are recurring recruitment problems with training and retaining sufficient numbers of professional carers for the elderly and for pre-school children (Wrede et al, 2008; Danmarks Radio, 2018). Given these profound changes, the question arises as to how to describe these changes and their effects upon care.

A convenient term that has emerged to describe these trends is 'care crisis'. The 'care crisis' concept was first introduced two decades ago by US sociologists (Phillips and Benner, 1994; Hochschild, 1995). The use of the term 'crisis' signals a derangement of matters, which can be thought of as relating to arrangements, decisions and beliefs (Wolin, 1969: 1080). While 'care crisis' can be seen as a useful shorthand for a wide gamut of trends, there are also risks in simply using a general, aggregate term and transferring an Anglo–American framing of care crisis into a different context. Scientific terms emerge in a specific milieu and academic disciplines, including terms describing care. Any care operates within its own unique welfare regimes. Hence, I decided to dig deeper and examine the original framing of a care crisis. By doing so, I position myself within the feminist tradition of self-reflexivity advocated by theorists such as Donna Haraway (1988) and Sandra Harding (1986). As the German sociologist Gudrun-Axeli Knapp has taught us, analytical concepts do not always travel easily across culturally and politically different contexts (2005)[2] and in this particular case, the concept travels too easily but may be misleading in the new environment of Nordic welfare regimes.

The concept of 'care crisis' is both a political and a scientific concept. It is used in various milieus, from policy debates to feminist care studies. It called attention to shortcomings in care as a result of changes in families and in the nature of the US welfare state (Phillips and Benner, 1994; Hochschild, 1995). The 'care crisis' discourse has travelled to other parts of the world, including the Nordic countries (Wrede et al, 2008; Isaksen, 2010) and Europe (Saraceno, 1997). Recently, the US feminist philosopher Nancy Fraser has called attention to the way in which a care crisis relates to a deeper crisis in capitalism and its current form of financialised capitalism (Fraser, 2016). The 'care crisis' concept has now diffused widely (Tronto, 2013; Lorey, 2015; Cottam, 2018; Jørgensen, 2019; Austrian Scholars of Care, 2020; The Care Collective, 2020).

In this chapter, I examine this scientific discourse on care crisis from a particular position and context as a feminist raised in a Nordic context. I am not studying this care crisis discourse as an outsider as I have used a similar term, 'care squeeze' (Dahl et al, 2011), in previous work. My analysis is a second-order analysis using a Foucault-inspired discourse analysis to analyse scientific texts as a form of data. I draw upon the discursive policy approach, 'What's the problem represented to be' (WPR), advocated by the Canadian-Australian political scientist Carol Bacchi (1999, 2009) in order to obtain a critical perspective upon this framing.[3] I will identify how the problem of a 'care crisis' is framed scientifically, applying a scaled-down version of the WPR approach. WPR directs our attention to particular ways of seeing and understanding social and political problems of care, to the silences in problem representations and their effects upon those researching Nordic welfare states and in other contexts. Based on an analysis of key care crisis texts, I will argue that the notion of a care crisis silences important aspects and that we need to revise the 'care crisis' concept if it is to be used in the Nordic context.

I will therefore offer a reading of a selection of key scientific texts on the care crisis, also using synonyms such as 'care deficit' (Hochschild, 1995) and 'care gap' (Fraser, 2016). In Nordic care research, there have been continuous discussions about threats to care but without using the notion of 'crisis' (see Dahl, 1997). The threats identified have been within formalised care work, for example, modernisation as rationalisation (Wærness, 1987; Jensen, 1992; Michaeli, 1995), bureaucratisation of care (Hamran 1996; Dahl, 2017) and the academisation of care professions (Martinsen, 1994; Eriksen, 1995; Johansson, 2001). Although this research has contributed important insights, it will not be discussed here. Rather, my focus will be on a sample of key Anglo-American scientific texts that have framed the 'care crisis' as the dominant understanding, also within a Nordic, social-democratic welfare regime – and elsewhere. Using the notion of 'hegemony' from Italian theorist Antonio Gramsci (1971), the Anglo-American understanding of the care crisis has become hegemonic, that is, performing a kind of discursive imperialism.

This chapter starts with a section on methodology. It then proceeds to the representation of the care crisis in the selected scientific texts, followed by a fourth section describing some of the silencing produced by this paradigm of a care crisis. In the fifth section, I discuss the discursive effects of this representation of the care crisis and possible alternative framings relevant to the Nordic context. Finally, I conclude by proposing that we rethink the concept of a care crisis.

Methodology and my position

By naming something, we create its existence (Wittgenstein, 1989). Without thinking and language, the care crisis would not be visible as a political problem. We need to pay attention, of course, to that which is articulated, but we also need to highlight that which is unthought and unsymbolised (Whitford, 1991). Thinking and language produce the terms of reference within which groups articulate their positions, bringing certain forms of social relationship into existence and silencing others (Foucault, 1978, 1980). I use the verb 'silencing' instead of the noun 'silence' to denote that silencing is an ongoing process rather than a state of affairs (Bacchi and Dahl, 2012; Dahl, 2017).

In my delimitation of the scientific field, I apply a broad notion of 'crisis' that invokes the term 'crisis' or its synonyms. My sole criteria have been the centrality of the texts within this tradition as well as whether this problem representation has developed over time. I have selected the most prominent researchers within the Anglo-American context: Phillips (1994), Hochschild (1995, 2001), Isaksen et al (2008) and recent texts by Fraser (2016) and Williams (2018), scholars who also identify several intersecting crises. Although this is a small sample, my selection of them is strategic: the selected texts introduce the concept, or they are the most important and influential within this field, or they add a crucial nuance to the original concept. I have delimited this scientific field, but I am well aware that other delimitations of it are possible. It is an attempt to view the 'care crisis' as a particular articulation of a problem in – and about – care as well as the silencing that invariably accompanies such problem articulations. Every scientific statement that intends to shed light on a problem will create its own shadows. Both the light and the shadows need to be explored.

I inhabit a double position as an insider to this scientific approach while simultaneously trying to position myself as an outsider in order to retrieve neglected insights and/or gain new ones. However, one of the insights from Foucault is that we cannot escape existing discourses, which makes becoming an outsider an impossibility. The most we can hope for is a kind of productive estrangement from existing discourses. I have researched gender and Nordic elder care in an era of neoliberalising and New Public Management. My research experience thus frames my analysis (Dahl, 2017), and I will return to this issue of reflexivity and the need to find ways to deconstruct the existing problem representation.

This chapter should not be seen as a review of the existing literature on 'care crisis'. Instead, it is a discourse analysis inspired by Michel Foucault and his call to study forms of knowledge and rationalities. By doing so, I also bring my epistemological position to work in reading scientific texts and I hope to achieve an alienation from the existing scientific discourse and its framing of the scientific problem in a particular way (Sandberg and Alvesson, 2011). More specifically, I draw upon the discursive policy analysis of Carol Bacchi (Bacchi, 1999, 2009; Bacchi and Goodwin, 2016). Bacchi works backwards in her WPR approach: from the policy solutions suggested in the texts to their representation of the policy problem. Identifying a problem representation is a difficult task, as it requires a dual process of familiarising oneself with the scientific literature closely, and then alienating oneself from the same scientific vocabulary, premises and understandings. Bacchi's discursive policy analysis involves seven steps (Bacchi, 2009; Bacchi and Goodwin, 2016): (1) What is the problem represented to be? (2) What assumptions underlie this representation of the problem? (3) How has this representation come about? (4) What is left unproblematic in this representation? (5) What effects are produced? (6) How/where has this representation of the 'problem' been produced – and how could it be disrupted? (7) Self-reflexivity, that is, how is my own analysis itself a representation of the problem?

For pragmatic reasons, I only consider some of the steps and modify them to fit my aim. I consider three main questions in my analysis: (1) How is the problem of a care crisis represented in the texts? And what is its extension, does it change and which kinds of assumptions is it based upon?[4] (This question combines steps 1 and 2 in Bacchi's approach and adds a historical element to the way the care crisis has been presented as a problem.) (2) What is seen, and particularly, what is not seen (silencing)? (Dahl, 2000, 2017; Bacchi, 2009). (This is similar to step 4 in Bacchi's approach.) (3) What are the effects of this problem representation for the Nordic welfare states, and can we disrupt or replace it with an alternative, scientific representation of a care crisis? (This contains elements of steps 5 and 6 in Bacchi's approach.) Through this critical analysis, I identify the dominant way in which the care crisis has been framed and seek to identify possibly suppressed elements, elements that have been silenced in the contemporary and/or the original texts. Silence operates in any text, neither as an opposite or outside, but as something within, which can be identified through meticulous analyses (Foucault, 1978; Haug et al, 1987; Dahl, 2012, 2017). Silencing refers to not seeing something as scientific discourses enable something to become visible and spoken about, and vice versa. In this analysis of three major questions, I also draw upon my former work (Dahl, 2000, 2011).

Instead of analysing policy texts as does Bacchi, I treat the scientific literature as empirical text data. I have read them backwards genealogically, starting with the most recent texts and then gradually moving backwards to the early formulations. I then analysed these data, applying the three questions in the previous paragraph, adapted to my research agenda. As a result, my analysis differs from Bacchi's, as my material consists of purely research-oriented texts without any kind of policy solution suggested. In this way, I cannot work backwards from solutions, as suggested by Bacchi. Instead, I identify and analyse the way in which the care crisis is articulated in the scientific texts. Identifying the problem representations is a way of reflecting upon, and eventually questioning, the received wisdom (Sandberg and Alvesson, 2011: 39). Although this is a rather ambitious enterprise, my ambition is more modest. I seek to pose questions regarding some of the key assumptions and silences in the framing of the care crisis.

Representations of the care crisis

The scientific application of a 'care crisis' concept began with two texts written in 1994 and 1995 by two US sociologists: Susan S. Phillips (1994) and Arlie R. Hochschild (1995). Later on, the notion of a 'care crisis' was extended from it being a strictly US-centred problem to a global one, with Hochschild's concept of 'global care chains' (Hochschild, 2001; Isaksen et al, 2008). This global focus continued in writings by the US philosopher Nancy Fraser (2016) and the British sociologist Fiona Williams (2018), who linked the care crisis to other global crises. In the following, I focus on these six core texts.

Although the representation of a care crisis changes over time in its Anglo-American version, there is a scientific framing of the care crisis across these six texts. The framing is that of an economistic model of the supply and demand for care, where there is an imbalance between the need for care personnel and the supply; that is, there is a scarcity of care that can be provided nationally and globally in an economistic model of care.

In her classic text from 1995, Hochschild describes the rising needs of care and a decreasing supply that creates a deficit of care in the private and public spheres:

> recent trends in the United States have expanded the need for care
> while contracting the supply of it. This has created a 'care deficit' in

both private and public life. In private life, the care deficit is most palpable in families where working mothers, married and single, lack sufficient help from partners or kin. ... In public life, the care deficit can be seen in government cuts in funds for services for poor mothers, the disabled, the mentally ill, and the elderly. In reducing the financial deficit, legislators add to the 'care deficit'. (Hochschild, 1995: 332)

The increasing need for care relates to changes in the nuclear family and in women's increasing labour market participation, whereas the decreasing supply of care providers is related to welfare state retrenchment (offloading care to families and communities) and a demanding labour market (Hochschild, 1995: 333–336). This picture of an imbalance between the supply and demand for care can also be identified in another early text, that of Phillips (1994). Instead of considering care in the family, she directs her gaze towards professional care in various institutions (such as health and education). Phillips detects an imbalance between what welfare ('caregiving') professionals see as their main task (the needs of care) and their possibilities of providing this within the framework of a care industry:

There is a crisis of caring for persons that cuts across the boundaries of the helping professions. Patients in hospitals feel depersonalized and processed, students suffer from inadequate attention, clients wonder if therapists really care about them. ... Caregivers are rewarded for efficiency, technical skill, and measurable results, while their concern, attentiveness, and human engagement go unnoticed within their professional organizations and institutions. (Phillips, 1994: 1)

In a bureaucratic system – public as well as private – suffused with rationality and neutrality, professional carers run into the dangers of 'depersonalization and disengagement' (Phillips, 1994: 6). The framing of a care crisis as one of lack of fit between supply and demand is applied in two different US settings: that of unpaid, family-based care work in the case of Hochschild, and that of professional care by Phillips (although Phillips has a more qualitative element as well). One could also see this representation as one of there being a sufficient number of 'hands' (carers), as in the case of Hochschild, or a case of suitable, attentive hands for care as described by Phillips with her notion of a 'crisis in care'. Although the care crisis seems to be framed in two different ways (by Hochschild and Phillips), Hochschild also includes qualitative and emotional elements in her typology of four different care models. The four models are called 'traditional', 'postmodern', 'cold-modern' and 'warm-modern'. Whereas the traditional model relies on the married male breadwinner with a homemaking wife/mother who cares for the children, and the sick and the elderly parent, the postmodern model relies upon a dual-breadwinner model where women 'do it all' without additional help from either spouse or paid carers. The cold–modern models refers to impersonal institutions[5] such as those described by Phillips (1994), and this contrasts with the warm–modern model, an ideal of care, where 'institutions provide some care of the young and elderly, while men and women join equally in providing private care as well' and which includes human engagement with those in need of care (Hochschild, 1995: 332). The warm–modern model is an ideal type of care that has not yet 'arrived'.

Empirically, Hochschild argues that the US is moving from a traditional to a postmodern model that legitimates the care deficit (Hochschild, 1995: 338). Here she describes a societal way of tackling the care crisis, where care needs are questioned and rewritten in a disguise of 'postmodern stoicism'. Care needs are neglected or reduced in order to fit the available care, using concepts such as 'self-care'. The care deficit is transformed from a social issue to a psychological issue, a matter of finding individual strategies to tackle the shortcomings in care that inevitably arise due to stressful jobs, unemployment, family crisis or illness (Hochschild, 1995: 339–340).

The more recent texts also frame a care crisis as that of supply and demand within a political economy. Williams (2018) and Isaksen et al (2008) see the care crisis in the Global North as leading to a care crisis in the Global South. Migrating care workers provide a partial solution to the care deficit of the Global North through their participation in the global care chain. This chain is defined as 'a series of personal links between people across the globe based on paid and unpaid work of caring' (Hochschild, 2001: 131).

Although global care chains ameliorate the care crisis in one country, they simultaneously erode social solidarities in the Global South and have negative, emotional effects upon the migrating mothers and their children left behind (Isaksen et al, 2008; Williams, 2018). New care crises are created in less wealthy parts of the world, such as Eastern Europe, the Philippines and India. Hence, 'the [care] markets of the North are indirectly eroding the social solidarities of the South' (Isaksen et al, 2008: 419).

Also, the most recent scientific texts describe a deficit of care. The care crisis is related to capitalism (Isaksen et al, 2008; Fraser, 2016; Williams, 2018), a specific form of capitalism and austerity measures (Fraser, 2016), to the commodification of care (Fraser, 2016; Williams, 2018) and to the growth in global migration (Isaksen et al, 2008; Williams, 2018). The migration crisis is seen as closely related to the care crisis (Isaksen et al, 2008; Williams, 2018).

Taking her point of departure in the media discussions of a care crisis in the US, Fraser (2016) detects a global care crisis that emanates from a contradiction in capitalism per se between production and reproduction (care), with boundary struggles about their respective role. For Fraser, capitalism 'freerides on – activities of provisioning, caregiving and interaction that produce and maintain social bonds, although it accords them no monetarized value and treats them as they were free' (Fraser, 2016: 101).

Following Fraser, in so far as the care crisis is embedded in capitalism, it is not a new phenomenon. For Fraser, the care crisis is indicative of a larger crisis in social reproduction, that is, of the social and cultural reproduction of our societies. It is not just about those who are vulnerable and dependent. Fraser rewrites the central contradiction as identified by Marx as a contradiction not between capital and labour, but between capital and care. This contradiction intensifies in capitalism's newest form, financialised capitalism,[6] and leads to struggles over care. The care crisis, therefore, is about 'externalizing care work onto families and communities' at the same time as capitalism 'diminished their capacity to perform it' (Fraser, 2016: 103). The care crisis relates to three other crises: that of capitalism per se, and political and ecological crises. Fraser adds to the existing literature on the care crisis by offering a historical, comparative, political–economic account that identifies the current crisis as related to a particular form of capitalism, state strategy and gender relations.

Taking her point of departure in four intersecting crises – care, capitalism, migration and ecology – Williams (2018) applies a political-economy approach together with a care ethical approach. Like Fraser, Williams is concerned about justice. In her view, global capitalism creates a global wage gap that makes it attractive for some to migrate, but compelling these migrating mothers to become emotionally amputated (leaving their children at home) (Williams, 2018: 417). The migration of these women thereby produces new care deficits in the extended care chain. The migration crisis is not sufficiently understood, nor is it taken sufficiently seriously as a social and political problem. Writing within a global sustainability discourse, and adapting the language of Polanyi, migration and capitalism turn people into 'fictitious commodities', where care is no longer sustainable. Williams argues that the 'commodification of care has led to its devaluation across the globe' (2018: 555), a line of argument also advanced by Fraser (2016).

Summarising, there is a basic problem representation that changes slightly over time, with common assumptions about the origin and dynamics of the care crisis. Across the texts, the care crisis is seen as having been ignored by the political system. This imbalance between the need for care and the available resources to provide care threatens the foundations of our society. The representation is one of accountancy, with the notion of 'resources' invoking a scenario of financial resources and hands/carers. There is an attention to the number of available carers and the number of children in need of care, thereby enforcing a division of the world into two mutually exclusive groups (and identities): those in need of care and those giving care.

Two major changes take place in the scientific discourse when a national care crisis is related to the occurrence of global care chains (Hochschild,

2001; Isaksen et al, 2008), and the care crisis is related to other crises (Fraser, 2016; Williams, 2018). One is that the care crisis now extends itself from a national to a global scale. The care crisis is identified in a US context, but it extends to a global one through the introduction of a political-economic perspective where some countries provide care labourers for others. The change from a national to a global perspective adds new causal factors to the crisis, such as capitalism, especially financialised capitalism, and inserts migration patterns into the original theories of 'changing family patterns' and 'retrenching welfare states'. More is going on than women entering the labour market and welfare states adopting neoliberalist reforms with/ without retrenchment.

This framing of 'hands' as the basic unit of care thereby aggregates needs for care from an individual to a societal level. There is also an assumption of family-based care as the most prevalent and ideal form of care. Kinship care becomes the basic kind of care. In this ideal of care, there is a negative view of the commodification of care that might delegitimise any form of care chains.[7] This critical view has implications for the view of care chains and the care chains created by professionals in hospitals, nursing homes and kindergartens, which are local rather than global. This problem representation turns professional care into something less desirable than family-based, non-commodified care. The assumption of simple identities of giving or receiving care is also problematic as it reduces the complexity of care, shifting needs and multiple identities. Such simplifications and dichotomisations have been criticised within the care literature (Tronto, 1991; Beasley and Bacchi, 2007), in that they point out our interdependence, vulnerability and complex identities. Let us therefore move on to identify some of the silencing processes that can be identified in the analysed texts.

Silence and silencing

There are many silences in the texts, not all of which can be uncovered (Dahl, 2012, 2017). Identifying silencing is a difficult enterprise and should not be confused with the researcher describing what she would have liked to have seen in the text. Rather, the silencing takes place within the text. Here I will focus upon the silencing that I have identified in most of the texts in some cases, and in a few cases in all the texts. Here I want to focus upon the beliefs – or logics – which pervade these scientific texts.

All of the texts refer to a care crisis. One of the beliefs in the representation of the 'crisis of care' problem is that of identifying the needs of particular groups, and as a corollary, the idea that these needs can be aggregated to a macro level, that is, the social system. However, counting is a way of ignoring differences. It is an intellectual 'coercion' brought about via the socialisation of children – and adults – when we are taught to count properly (Stone,

2018). The care crisis frames all needs as similar, such as the needs of 'all pre-school children' to be cared for. However, this representation silences the differences between the children (or for that matter, other groups) and the different kinds of care that these children require. The intangibles of the world are simplified, fragmented and aggregated into the figure of the 'needy child', the 'needy elderly' or 'the challenged person'. Needs are simplified and homogenised, thereby neglecting those children who have difficulties performing as competent, resilient and flexible children or of those elderly who are too weak to adhere to the norm of 'active ageing'. By silencing differences within groups, a whole world of care needs and wishes are neglected.

Another silencing process relates to the neglect of different groups in need of care. Originally, there was an attention to the care of children, as in the text by Hochschild (1995). Except for Phillips' text that is forgotten in the most recent contributions to the literature, this focus upon children continues, thereby producing a silencing of other groups, such as elder care. Although elder care has been at the forefront of the political agenda for decades, the main feminist theorisation on the care crisis has continued to silence elder care, despite some exceptions (for example, Isaksen, 2010). However, the framing of care as centred on childcare necessarily neglects differences in the ways in which the silencing of different target groups operates between welfare regimes, different state strategies and translations of neoliberalising in various institutional contexts. As a comparative study of European elder care has shown, there are major differences within Europe in the kind and extent of care provided for the fragile elderly. Whereas some welfare states have expanded their state-financed elder care, others have carried out reforms and still others proceeded with retrenchment (Ranci and Pavolini, 2013). The profound differences in welfare regimes cannot be accounted for in this framing of a care crisis that relies on a general, systemic account concerned with numbers. This silencing of key categories hides the historical development of the different welfare states and their different translations of the processes of neoliberalising.

Another important silencing concerns the work of professional carers and institutional care. These issues, originally raised by Phillips (1994), have been overlooked in the more recent care crisis literature. The representation of the care crisis avoids attending to professional care and how the care crisis unfolds in either market-based or state-financed institutions of pre-school care, after-school activities, nursing homes, home help or hospitals. The texts focus their attention largely on family-based care and on care-giving work commodified in capitalist markets, as if all care were still primarily performed within the confines of the home. This neglect of the institutional settings not only leads to a skewed analysis; it is simply anachronistic. Capitalism and commodification may make for bad-quality care or poor working conditions for carers, but we lack elaborations of why the commodification of care is necessarily bad in a situation of increasing division of labour, and especially women's increasing paid labour.[8]

Although the texts generally apply a gender perspective, they silence changing masculinities. Men are generally not seen, or if they are seen, it is in a context of their evasion of care responsibilities, especially in the earlier texts (Hochschild, 1995). However, much has happened since the 1990s. Within research on masculinity, there is an ongoing discussion about changing masculinities. On the one hand, there are researchers arguing that a business-oriented masculinity has become dominant, whereas others argue that a caring masculinity has become more common. The Australian sociologist Raewyn Connell (2005) has argued that contemporary masculinities are plural, hierarchical and dynamic, while the Norwegian sociologist Øystein G. Holter argues that men – or some groups of men – increasingly stress their fatherhood and caring responsibilities, at least towards their children. We are witnessing the rise of a caring model of masculinity, that of 'involved fathers', at least in the Nordic countries (Holter, 2003; Farstad and Stefansen, 2015), and these fathers are having an impact upon the care of small children. Having identified a silencing of different care needs, different groups in need of care as well as professional care, men and changing gender identities, let me now move on to the effects of this framing.

The effects of the prevalent care crisis representation

In Bacchi's approach, any given problem representation has various effects (Bacchi, 2009: 15–18). Here I focus only upon the discursive effects for care researchers. The question here is: What does this framing do to us as researchers who study and live in Nordic welfare states? What is the impact of this type of framing on the global community of care scholars? These questions open up an increasing awareness and reflexivity about our own positioning as Nordic care scholars, and the analytical concepts and premises with which we operate.

One of the assumptions in the dominant framing of the Anglo-American-inspired 'care crisis' is the idea that the crisis stems from insufficient resources. This kind of representation will most likely tend to lead researchers into a preoccupation with statistics and budgets, literally with 'counting hands'. We become preoccupied with budget cuts and retrenchment. However, as I have shown, retrenchment can take place even in the midst of a non-retrenching welfare state in economic terms (Dahl, 2005). Being attentive to the inputs and outputs is important for understanding the nature of a system, how it constructs 'needs' and how it 'delivers' the care given. However, such a framing leads us to overlook what happens *inside* care in the welfare state: the black box of the discursive governance of care and of care provided by care professionals in institutions. Here, a transnational discourse of neoliberalising may end up clashing with the specificities of the Nordic welfare states. Each individual welfare state responds to and translates this neoliberal discourse differently, having potentially different impacts upon the care provided. The dominant framing of a care crisis reduces everything to determining whether or not 'care' is being provided. But 'care' has a qualitative dimension. What about *good* care? What is good care in an institutional setting in welfare states that are ostensibly governed by universalism and the rule of law (e.g. impartiality)? Such questions cannot be asked when the 'care crisis' framework is concerned only with the 'amount' of care as an indicator.[9] Neither does this representation give us tools to discuss professional care work in a broad sense, such as the conditions for providing care with empathy. This does not mean that issues of resources (money and time) are irrelevant. However, discussion of these issues needs to be supplemented by a discussion of the emotions and knowledge connected to care. Emotions are mentioned by Hochschild (1995), Phillips (1994) and Isaksen et al (2008). However, emotions are not systematically related to the different kinds of knowledge that are necessary to provide good care and to the privileging of some forms of knowledge in public policies. In feminist sociology, care is a triad of hand, heart and head, where thinking, doing and feeling are important dimensions (Leira, 1994).

Another discursive effect of the hegemonic understanding of the care crisis is the sidestepping of issues of rights. Focusing upon the imbalance between demands for care and availability of care, and of fulfilling needs, means that issues of rights to receive and give care are not discussed. Precisely these issues have been raised by feminist scholars (Knijn and Kremer, 1997). They have focused on the balance between those in need of care and those providing care, the balance between informal, family-based care and formalised (paid) care, and the balance between cash services and cash for care paid by welfare states to either the person in direct need of care or their family. Hence, I suggest that one of the questions in feminist theorising, and theorising about care and the care crisis, is: Who should have which kinds of rights and to what? Although we cannot reduce the care crisis in the Nordic welfare states, assuming such a crisis exists, to an issue of assigning rights (and its inherent individualistic bias), the Nordic welfare regimes already possess a strong tradition of thinking in terms of rights to receive care.

There are also effects of the early framing by which different forms of a care crisis are distinguished; however, these four different ideal types have not yet received much attention. In the 'postmodern ideal type' (Hochschild, 1995), for instance, care needs are downsized and rewritten, thereby legitimising a permanent care crisis. We might consider whether this particular ideal type fits the Nordic welfare states today, where care needs are being reformulated from that of helping and caring to a more indirect form of 'coaching'[10] the elderly and challenged people into a new ideal of self-motivated activity, active ageing and self-help with notions of 'self-care' and 're-ablement' (Dahl, 2012, 2017; Dahl et al, 2015). Policy ideals of 'self-care' and 're-ablement' are frequently articulated as means of enhancing the autonomy of the elderly. However, pursuit of these ideals also results in a change – and reduction – in the kind of care provided by the municipalities on behalf of the state from compensatory care to self-care by the elderly. Such policies also potentially punish the fragile elderly who are made to feel that they are morally lacking because they cannot perform 'self-care', that is, adhere to the ideal of 'active ageing'.

Finally, we could ask what a problem representation that focuses upon commodification of care as detrimental can bring to us as feminist scholars researching and theorising the Nordic welfare states? In the texts by Fraser and Williams, commodification of care is problematised as undesirable and bringing misrecognition along with it. Misrecognition is about cultural domination, non-recognition and disrespect (Fraser, 1997a, 2003): about not being seen and heard (Thompson, 2006), and not taken into account in social interaction. This is a plea to reflect upon misrecognition of care-giving work and its causes, especially whether capitalism works together with a gendered system of valorisation, which creates hierarchies of work and knowledges. So is commodification necessarily bad in itself? Or is it commodification of care together with patriarchal values of care that are undesirable? Commodification refers to three kinds of societal processes: (1) care going into the market (between individuals or between an individual and a private firm); (2) care going into the state, that is, tax financing of universally accessible care; and (3) hybrid care, where care financed by the state is outsourced to be provided by the market. However, commodification hardly ever occurs alone but in a complex interplay with other societal and politically engineered processes. In the Nordic welfare states, care has to a large extent become a state responsibility and the state has been involved in its professionalising. This has not ended the discussion about the misrecognition of care (Dahl, 2004, 2009, 2010; Hoppania, 2015). Research shows that commodifying care by the state and state strategies to professionalise care work have not led to a feminist nirvana of recognition, despite the fact that care work in the Nordic welfare states has gained more recognition compared to other welfare regimes (Dahl, 2004, 2009). Despite its elements of women-friendliness, the state has reproduced gendered values of productive versus unproductive work, and in doing so reproduced misrecognition. This is not to place blame on the commodification of care, but on gendered discourses of what counts as valuable (Dahl, 2010).

Conclusion

The notion of a 'care crisis' was 'born in the USA', with its liberal welfare regime, rampant neoliberalism and New Public Management reforms. This is hardly a coincidence. However, the 'care crisis' has become a fast-travelling concept in feminist science and in the media. Concepts are not innocent, and although some may travel easily, they may be misleading in a new environment (Knapp, 2005). Travelling concepts bring along a problem representation that I have analysed using Bacchi's discursive policy analysis and applying it to scientific texts. Analysing these core texts describing an ostensible 'care crisis', I have identified a representation of a care crisis as an economistic model of supply of and demand for care, tallying up statistics about needs, ignoring important differences in care needs within groups and with an analytical attention on children to the exclusion of the elderly. The care crisis was originally attached to a 'retrenchment of the welfare state' and 'changes in the nuclear family'. This framing was slightly modified when the care crisis was reformulated as a global care system depending on migration. Capitalism, and a particular form of capitalism, and migration were added as factors behind the global – and national – care crisis.

The framing is premised upon simple identities of care-givers and care-receivers, thereby ignoring the complexity of care. The representation of a care crisis also revealed silencing of elder care, neglect of professional care and overlooking of the positive role of caring men. It also produced effects that would cause us to neglect issues of what constitutes good care, the role of knowledge and the relationships between needs and rights.

The notion of a 'care crisis' turns our attention towards aspects of reproduction and the care that have often been neglected – care that is necessary for our continued existence and for living good lives. However, we found neglected insights in the literature on care crisis that deserve further study. Phillips' insights on the challenges for professionals in the industry of caring have been forgotten by those researchers deploying a global political-economic perspective. The insights from Hochschild on different ideals of care, and especially notions of postmodern care and cold-modern care, could be relevant to the Nordic welfare regimes and merit further exploration. Also, turning our attention to silences within Nordic research on care, it seems that informal care within families for the elderly or challenged have not received much attention, and would also merit further exploration.

The representation of a care crisis in its current form involves assumptions, important silences and serious, discursive effects upon us as care researchers. We need to turn our attention to the silenced issues of the current framing of a care crisis. At the very least, we can start reflecting upon how to revise the concept of a care crisis generally, and specifically, to make it applicable in the Nordic welfare regimes.

Notes

[1] I use the notion of 'neoliberalising' as a verb instead of neoliberalisation. By using a verb instead of a noun, I want to stress that it is a political process and not deterministic, and that neoliberalising is a field of struggles (Dahl, 2017).

[2] Recently, an anthropologist has argued that the concept of 'care' itself has a 'specific, cultural freight' stemming from its Anglo-American heritage, for example by using the analytical distinction of caring for and caring about (Buch, 2015).

[3] Bacchi applies the notion of 'problematization' (Bacchi, 2009: xii) inspired by Foucault.

[4] By assumptions, Bacchi refers to a kind of archeological analysis suggested by Foucault, paying attention to the way objects and subjects are constituted as well as the dominant rationalities (Bacchi, 2009: 5).

[5] The cold-modern model Hochschild refers to care performed in state-financed – and provided – care in the former socialist countries of Eastern Europe.

[6] Financialised capitalism refers to the increasing role of finance capital in capitalism. Finance capital, or financialisation, is the way non-financial corporations are integrated more deeply into liberalised capital markets (Horton, 2019). An example from the UK is care homes being bought by private equity firms and other investment funds (Horton, 2019: 2).

[7] The term 'commodification' is complex as it is about care becoming paid work, but it can become so in the marketplace, in the state and in the hybrid of outsourcing state-financed care to the market.

[8] The neglect of institutional care raises the recurring issue of whether women's work is poorly paid because it is gendered, or whether it becomes gendered because it is poorly paid.

[9] This analysis of the six texts doesn't take account of former and other work of the authors. This is naturally unfair towards Nancy Fraser, who in her earlier work (Fraser, 1997b) discussed different ideals of care, for example her universal care-giver model.

[10] The notion of 'coaching' is taken from the Danish sociologists Margareta Järvinen and Nanna Mik-Meyer (Järvinen and Mik-Meyer, 2012).

References

Austrian Scholars of Care (2020) 'Groszputz! Care nach Corona neu gestalten', Available from: https://care-macht-meht.com [accessed 5 November 2020].

Bacchi, C. (1999) *Women, Policy and Politics: The Construction of Policy Problems*, London: SAGE.

Bacchi, C. (2009) *What's the Problem Represented to Be?* French Forests: Pearson.

Bacchi, C. and Dahl, H.M. (2012) 'Silencing: Inside/outside', unpublished manuscript.

Bacchi, C. and Goodwin, S. (2016) *Poststructural Policy Analysis: A Guide to Practice*, London: Palgrave.

Beasley, C. and Bacchi, C. (2007) 'Envisaging a new politics for an ethical future: Beyond trust, care and generosity – towards an ethics of "social flesh"', *Feminist Theory*, 8(3): 279–298.

Buch, E. (2015) 'Anthropology of aging and care', *Annual Review of Anthropology*, 44: 277–293.

The Care Collective (2020) *The Care Manifesto*, London: Verso.

Clarke, J. and Newman, J. (1997) *The Managerial State*, London: SAGE.

Connell, R. (2005) 'Masculinities and globalisation' in M.A. Zinn et al (eds) *Gender Through the Prism of Difference*, Oxford: Oxford University Press, pp 36–48.

Cottam, H. (2018) *Radical Help: How Can We Remake the Relationship Between Us & Revolutionize the Welfare State*, London: Virago Little Brown.

Dahl, H.M. (1997) 'Mellem kærlighed og arbejde – omsorgsteori: Traditioner og centrale temaer', *Kvinder, Køn og Forskning*, 6(2): 56–65.

Dahl, H.M. (2000) *Fra kitler til eget tøj – Diskurser om professionalisme, omsorg og køn*, PhD thesis, Aarhus: Politica.

Dahl, H.M. (2004) 'A view from the inside: Recognition and redistribution in the Nordic welfare state from a gender perspective', *Acta Sociologica*, 47(4): 325–337.

Dahl, H.M. (2005) 'A changing ideal of care in Denmark: A different form of retrenchment?' in H.M. Dahl and T.R. Eriksen (eds) *Dilemmas of Care: Continuity and Change*, Aldershot: Ashgate, pp 47–61.

Dahl, H.M. (2009) 'New Public Management, care and struggles about recognition', *Critical Social Policy*, 29(4): 634–654.

Dahl, H.M (2010) 'An old map of state feminism and an insufficient recognition of care', *NORA*, 18(3): 152–166.

Dahl, H.M. (2011) 'Who can be against quality?' in C. Ceci, K. Björnsdottir and M.E. Purkis (eds) *Home, Care and Practices: Critical Perspectives on Frailty*, London: Routledge, pp 139–157.

Dahl, H.M. (2012) 'Tavshed som magt og afmagt', *Tidsskriftet Antropologi*, 33(66): 3–16.

Dahl, H.M. (2017) *Struggles in (Elderly) Care: A Feminist View*, London: Palgrave Macmillan.

Dahl, H.M., Keränen, M. and Kovalainen, A. (2011) 'Introduction', in H.M. Dahl, M. Keränen and A. Kovalainen (eds) *Europeanization, Care and Gender: Global Complexities*, London: Palgrave Macmillan, pp 1–17.

Dahl, H.M., Eskelinen, L. and Hansen, E.B. (2015) 'Co-existing principles of good elder care: Help-to-self-help and consumer-oriented care?' *The International Journal on Social Welfare*, 24(3): 287–295.

Dahl, H.M., Hansen, A.E., Hansen, C.S. and Kristensen, J.E. (2015) *Kamp og status: De lange linjer i børnehaveinstitutionens og pædagogprofessionens historie 1820 til 1915*, Copenhagen: UPress.

Danmarks Radio (2018) 'Ældreplejen mangler hænder: flertal kræver lynforhandlinger hos Thyra Frank', Available from: www.dr.dk/nyheder/politik/aeldreplejen-mangler-haender-flertal-kraever-lynforhandlinger-hos-thyra-frank [accessed 19 November 2020].

Eriksen, T.R. (1995) *Omsorg i forandring*, Copenhagen: Munksgaard.

Esping-Andersen, G. (1990) *The Three Worlds of Welfare Capitalism*, Cambridge: Polity Press.

Farstad, G.R. and Stefansen, K. (2015) 'Involved fatherhood in the Nordic context: Dominant narratives, divergent approaches', *NORMA: International Journal for Masculinity Studies*, 10(1): 55–70.

Foucault, M. (1978) *The History of Sexuality*, London: Penguin.

Foucault, M. (1980) *Power/Knowledge: Selected Interviews and Other Writings 1972–1977 by Michael Foucault*, London: Prentice Hall.

Fraser, N. (1997a) *Justice Interruptus*, New York: Routledge.

Fraser, N. (1997b) 'After the family wage: A postindustrialist thought experiment' in N. Fraser, *Justice Interruptus*, New York: Routledge.

Fraser, N. (2003) 'Social justice in the age of identity politics' in N. Fraser and A. Honneth (eds) *Redistribution or Recognition?* London: Verso, pp 7–108.

Fraser, N. (2016) 'Contradictions of capital and care', *New Left Review*, 100(July/August): 99–117.

Gramsci, A. (1971) *Selections from Prison Notebooks*, edited by Q. Hoare and G.N. Smith, London: Lawrence & Wishart.

Hamran, T. (1996) 'Effektivisering versus omsorgsansvar', *Kvinneforskning*, 2: 35–48.

Haraway, D. (1988) 'Situated knowledges: The science question in feminism and the privilege of perspective', *Feminist Studies*, 14(3): 575–599.

Harding, S. (1986) *The Science Question in Feminism*, Milton Keynes: Open University Press.

Haug, F., Althusser, L., Anderson, P., Eagleton, T., Jameson, F., Rose, J. et al (1987) 'Memory work', in F. Haug et al (eds) *Female Sexualisation*, London: Verso, pp 33–72.

Hernes, H. (1987) *Welfare State and Woman Power: Essays in State Feminism*, Oslo: Universitetsforlaget.

Hochschild, A.R. (1995) 'The politics of culture: Traditional, cold modern, post modern and warm modern ideals of care', *Social Politics: International Studies in Gender, State, and Society*, 2(3): 331–346.

Hochschild, A.R. (2001) 'Global care chains and emotional surplus value' in W. Hutton and A. Giddens (eds) *On the Edge: Living with Global Capitalism*, London: Vintage, pp 130–146.

Holter, Ø.G. (2003) *Can Men Do It? Men and Gender Equality: The Nordic Experience*, Copenhagen: TemaNord.

Hoppania, H. (2015) *Care as a Site for Political Struggles*, PhD thesis, Helsinki: Department of Political and Economic Studies, Helsinki University.

Horton, A. (2019) 'Financialization and non-disposable women: Real estate, debt and labour in the UK care homes', *Economy and Space*: 1–16. Available from: https://doi.org/10.1177/0308518X19862580 [accessed 2 July 2021].

Isaksen, L.W. (2010) 'Introduction' in L.W. Isaksen (ed) *Global Care Work: Gender and Migration in Nordic Societies*, Lund: Nordic Academic Press, pp 9–19.

Isaksen, L.W., Devi, U. and Hochschild, A.R. (2008) 'Global care crisis: A problem of capital, care chain or commons?', *American Behavioral Scientist*, 52(3): 405–425.

Järvinen, M. and Mik-Meyer, N. (2012) 'Indledning' in M. Järvinen and N. Mik-Meyer (eds) *At skabe en professionel*, Copenhagen: Hans Reitzel, pp 13–28.

Jensen, K. (1992) *Hjemlig omsorg i offentligt regi*, Oslo: Universitetsforlaget.

Johansson, S. (2001) *Den sociale omsorgens akademisering*, Stockholm: Liber.

Jørgensen, S.L. (2019) 'De fagprofessionelle, behovsfortolkning og legitimitet i ældreplejepolitikken', *Politica*, 51(2): 187–210.

Knapp, G. (2005) 'Race, class, gender: Reclaiming baggage in fast travelling theories', *European Journal of Women's Studies*, 12(3): 249–265.

Knijn, T. and Kremer, M. (1997) 'Gender and the caring dimension of welfare states: Toward inclusive citizenship', *Social Politics*, 4(3): 328–361.

Leira, A. (1994) 'The concept of caring: Loving, thinking, and doing', *Social Service Review*, 68(2): 185–201.

Lorey, I. (2015) *State of Insecurity: Government of the Precarious*, London: Verso.

Martinsen, K. (1994) *Fra Marx til Løgstrup: Om etik og sanselighed i sygeplejen*, Copenhagen: Munksgaard.

Meagher, G. and Szebehely, M. (2013) 'Four Nordic countries: Four responses to the international trend of marketization' in G. Meagher and M. Szebehely (eds) *Marketization in Nordic Elder care*, Stockholm: Department of Social Work, pp 241–283.

Michaeli, I. (1995) *Omsorg och rättvisa – ett dilemma*, Gävle: Meyers.

Phillips, S.S. (1994) 'Introduction' in S.S. Phillips and P. Benner (eds) *The Crisis of Care: Affirming and Restoring Caring Practices in the Helping Professions*, Washington, DC: Georgetown University Press, pp 1–15.

Phillips, S.S. and Benner, P. (eds) (1994) *The Crisis of Care: Affirming and Restoring Caring Practices in the Helping Professions*, Washington, DC: Georgetown University Press.

Ranci, C. and Pavolini, E. (2013) 'Reforms in long-term care policies in Europe: An introduction' in C. Ranci and E. Pavolini (eds) *Reforms in Long-Term Care Policies in Europe: Investigating Institutional Change and Social Impacts*, New York: Springer, pp 3–22.

Sandberg, J. and Alvesson, M. (2011) 'Ways of constructing research questions: Gap-spotting or problematization?' *Organization*, 18(1): 23–44.

Saraceno, C. (1997) *Family, Market and Community*, Paris: OECD.

Stone, D. (2018) 'The 2017 James Madison Award lecture: The ethics of counting', *PS: Political Science & Politics*, 51(1): 7–16.

Thompson, S. (2006) *The Political Theory of Recognition*, Cambridge: Polity.

Tronto, J. (1991) *Moral Boundaries: A Political Argument for an Ethic of Care*, New York: Routledge.

Tronto, J. (2013) *Caring Democracy: Markets, Equality, and Justice*, New York: New York University Press.

Vabø, M. and Szebehely, M. (2012) 'A caring state for all older people?', in A. Anttonen, L. Häikö and K. Stefasson (eds) *Welfare State, Universalism and Diversity*, Cheltenham: Edward Elgar, pp 212–43.

Wærness, K. (1987) 'On the rationality of caring', in A. Showstack Sassoon (ed) *Women and the State*, London: Hutchinson, pp 207–34.

Whitford, M. (1991) *Luce Irigaray: Philosophy in the Feminine*, London: Routledge.

Williams, F. (2018) 'Care: Intersections of scales, inequalities and crises', *Current Sociology*, 66(4): 547–61.

Wittgenstein, L. (1989) *Om vished*, Århus: Philosophia.

Wolin, S.S. (1969) 'Political theory as a vocation', *The American Political Science Review*, 63(4): 1062–1082.

Wrede, S., Henriksson, L., Høst, H., Johansson, S. and Dybbroe, B. (2008) 'Introduction: Care work and the competing rationalities of public policy' in S. Wrede, L. Henriksson, H. Høst, S. Johansson and B. Dybbroe (eds) *Care Work in Crisis: Reclaiming the Nordic Ethos of Care*, Lund: Studentlitteratur, pp 15–37.

3

Fraser's care crisis theory meets the Nordic welfare societies

Lise Lotte Hansen, Margunn Bjørnholt and Laura Horn

Introduction

The aim of this chapter is to place Nancy Fraser's care crisis concept in the Nordic welfare society context. Fraser has developed her discussion of the care crisis with a focus mainly on the Anglo-American model, that is, in societies very different from the Nordic welfare model regarding the organisation of reproductive work, gender equality policies and labour market regulation. In her broad framework, 'crisis of care' is 'best interpreted *as a more or less acute* expression of the social-reproductive contradictions of financialised capitalism' (Fraser, 2016: 99, emphasis added). In this chapter, we argue that her understanding of the role of reproductive work in capitalist societies today, as well as the idea of a deepening care crisis also makes sense in a discussion of Nordic societies. There is, however, a need to take into account the historically specific institutional configurations, policies and social practices that render the dynamics of care crisis in the Nordic welfare states different and variegated, but nonetheless fundamentally engender crisis tendencies that are becoming more and more visible.

Fraser's main argument is that reproductive work is rendered invisible, even though it constitutes a necessary 'background condition of possibility' for production (Fraser, 2016). This argument is not new. Feminist care theorists argue that care is at the core of any society (for example Tronto, 1993, 2013, 2017; Kittay, 1999). Feminist economists (Dalla Costa and James, 1975; Waring, 1988; Ferber and Nelson, 1993; Henderson, 1996; Folbre, 2001, among others) have argued that all production of economic value is based on unpaid work and resources whose value – and costs – are not reflected in the formal economy, and that the appropriation of unpaid work and unvalued resources is central to the accumulation of capital on a global scale (Mies, 1986). In her pioneering study on the role of unpaid work in a Nordic welfare state context, the Norwegian sociologist Kari Wærness (1978, 1984) argued that the (Norwegian) welfare state relied on women's unpaid care work. Fraser's contribution to this discussion lies in unambiguously linking the disregard and misrecognition of care to the sustainability of capitalism as a

39

system (Fraser, 2014). The invisibility of the dependency between production and reproduction has resulted in increasing pressure on both paid and unpaid care work in neoliberal capitalism. For now, the crisis is primarily a care crisis, but it will develop into a crisis *of* capitalism as such because the one-sided prioritizing of productive work and economic growth will destabilise reproductive processes, which are a condition for the existence of capitalist societies (Fraser, 2016; Bhattacharya, 2017).

> This peculiar relation of separation-cum-dependence-cum-disavowal is an inherent source of instability: on the one hand, capitalist economic production is not self-sustaining, but relies on social reproduction; on the other, its drive to unlimited accumulation threatens to destabilise the very reproductive processes and capacities that capital – and the rest of us – need. The effect over time, as we shall see, can be to jeopardise the necessary social conditions of the capitalist economy. (Fraser, 2016: 103)

With regard to applying Fraser's framework to the ongoing transformation of the Nordic welfare states, it is relevant to focus here on how these specific patterns emerge and manifest in a care crisis. Conceptually, this requires an understanding of the distinct and uneven *variegated* forms of welfare capitalism. Neoliberalism, or rather the process of neoliberalisation, constitutes a 'politically guided intensification of market rule and commodification' (Brenner et al, 2010: 184). This is a meaningful differentiation as it allows for investigation of the shared trajectories and specific manifestations of the care crisis in the Nordic welfare states that takes into account the specificities and commonalities of these developments.

In the Nordic welfare societies, a considerable share of care and reproductive work has been turned into paid work in the public sector. It still is (mainly) women's work, and it provides women with an income (Koren, 2012; Aslaksen and Koren, 2014). This is one of the reasons for talking about Nordic welfare societies as potentially 'women-friendly' (Hernes, 1987). Another reason is that welfare state services and social security have made it possible for women to combine motherhood, paid work and active citizenship, resulting in women getting a new bargaining position and a higher degree of equality (Christensen and Siim, 2001; see also Borchorst and Siim, 2010). Yet the contradictions of state-managed welfare systems in an overall context of increasingly financialised capitalism (Dowling, 2017) mean that care crisis tendencies are also present in Nordic societies. They become manifest as pressure on both paid and unpaid care work, as well as pressure on communities; manifest with regard to gender dimensions as well as other vectors of discrimination and oppression, such as ethnicity, race and age. It is important to consider that this is not only a problem regarding gender equality and respect for care workers, care-givers and care-receivers, but that these contradictions question the sustainability of the Nordic welfare societies in general.

In Fraser's discussion of the crisis of care, there is a latent hesitation to formulate strong answers to the question of how to resolve these contradictions. As the discussion of 'women-friendly' welfare states has shown, for many observers (and those participating in contemporary debates) the Nordic model appears as a best practice model – almost as a critical case that attempts to resolve the contradictions of capital and care. Like many US family researchers, Arlie R. Hochschild (1995), for instance, has been an admirer of the Nordic model of care, arguing that this 'warm-modern model' combines a market model with time to care.

This chapter contributes to these discussions by highlighting how the care crisis surfaces in Nordic welfare societies, and how Fraser's framework is fruitful for such an analysis; starting with the development of indicators of a care crisis and then discussing these in relation to changes in the Nordic welfare societies. As such, the chapter draws on a rereading and reworking of analyses from previous research projects. In the first part, we engage with core dimensions of care and gender equality in Fraser's care crisis concept, and in the Nordic welfare states, respectively. We summarise this conceptual discussion in a table outlining core indicators of care crisis dynamics. This juxtaposition is then followed by illustrations of care crisis dynamics in Denmark and Norway, drawing on the indicators developed earlier, and focusing on different spheres of social reproduction, namely financialisation, recognition of family and care work, and social struggles and resistance. The concluding reflections highlight the need for a historically and institutionally specific understanding of these transformative trajectories of the care crisis in the Nordic welfare states.

Engaging with Fraser's concepts of care crisis and social justice

Fraser's starting point is the way the capitalist system relies on social reproductive activities external to the economy:

> activities of provisioning, care-giving and interaction that produce and maintain social bonds, although it accords them no monetised value and treats them as if they were free. Variously called 'care', 'affective labour' or 'subjectivation', such activity forms capitalism's human subjects, sustaining them as embodied natural beings, while also constituting them as social beings, forming their habitus and the cultural ethos in which they move. The work of birthing and socialising the young is central to this process, as is caring for the old, maintaining households, building communities and sustaining the shared meanings, affective

dispositions and horizons of value that underpin social cooperation. (Fraser, 2016: 101)

All of these, predominantly unrecognised, devalued and unpaid, activities of social reproduction provide 'an indispensable background condition for the possibility of economic production in a capitalist society' (Fraser, 2016: 102). The fundamental contradiction that the formal economy relies on the use of unpaid care work as well as of the extraction and destruction of natural resources, both of which are treated as 'free', has been one of the main arguments of feminist economists and feminist theorists of care (Dalla Costa and James, 1975; Waring, 1988; Henderson, 1996; Folbre, 2001). Fraser's (2013) particular contribution lies in linking this critique to a broader analysis of (contemporary) capitalism and a theorisation of the relations between marketisation, social protection and emancipation. Crucially, in particular with regard to a focus on agency and emancipatory struggles, this systemic critique also expands on her previous work by arguing that there is a link between liberal feminism and neoliberalism (Fraser, 2009).

Fraser's framework shows that the contradiction between care and production is inherent in capitalism, and that the way in which this contradiction is resolved in historically specific regimes is linked to particular gender arrangements. She develops three regimes, with contemporary financialised capitalism constituting the most recent manifestation of these contradictions (Fraser, 2016: 104). This regime relies on the dual-earner model, in combination with a simultaneous disinvestment in social care. As Fraser argues (2016: 112):

> Globalizing and neoliberal, this regime promotes state and corporate disinvestment from social welfare, while recruiting women into the paid workforce—externalizing carework onto families and communities while diminishing their capacity to perform it. The result is a new, dualized organization of social reproduction, commodified for those who can pay for it and privatized for those who cannot, as some in the second category provide carework in return for (low) wages for those in the first.

The two-earner household has become a paradigmatic node in this regime. However, an overall falling wage share coupled with an increase in precarious employment is undermining the sustainability of this model. As households struggle to cover the costs of social reproduction, they are increasingly forced into debt to finance care and other aspects of social reproduction. Moreover, this regime is based on the lower social status of, and lower pay for, reproductive work. When money and paid work are everything, unpaid care work is almost invisible as a necessary activity for society; yet care work (unpaid *and* paid) creates and sustains our 'capacity to work' in the first place.

> And that means fashioning people with the 'right' attitudes, dispositions and values; abilities competences and skills. All told, people-making work supplies some fundamental preconditions – material, cultural, social – for human society in general and for capitalist production in particular. Without it, neither life nor labour power could be embodied in human beings. (Arruzza et al, 2018: 121)

It is crucial to emphasise here, as Fraser argues, that these contradictions are *not* accidental, but rather, 'have deep systemic roots in the structure of our social order ... not only in capitalism's current, financialised form but in capitalist society per se' (Fraser, 2016: 100). At the same time, social reproduction also includes 'non-commodified' zones, ideals, values, affective relations and practices with their own logic, engendered by care, mutual responsibility and solidarity (Fraser, 2014: 66). Feminist economists insist that this orientation to communities and love are fundamental to humankind and our societies (Bjørnholt and McKay, 2014). This highlights the relational power structures between production and reproduction; gendered understandings of various aspects of care work (paid and unpaid), and broader patterns of physical, affective and emotional labour that constitute the fabric of care that maintains societal processes. Social reproduction is therefore not only about caring for people, but includes caring for things, communities and the Earth (Tronto, 1993; 2013; Bjørnholt and McKay, 2014; Fraser, 2014; O'Hara, 2014; Bjørnholt, 2018).

For our analysis, we operationalise Fraser's care crisis concept into five dimensions, summarised in Table 3.1, each including a range of care crisis indicators. These dimensions stand in a dynamic relation to each other, with the first one outlining the overarching production – social reproduction dynamic in capitalist societies. This contradiction is fundamental to capitalist societies and 'surfaces' as a deepening care crisis in financialised capitalism, which threatens societal sustainability. We extract the core elements of Fraser's thinking, drawing on a broad range of her texts (Fraser, 2009, 2013, 2014, 2016) and another paper written in conjunction with Arruzza and Bhattacharya (Aruzza et al, 2018).

The freeriding, exploitation and undervaluation of care do not just go on without protest, they also produce conflicts and struggles. Social reproduction struggles are especially explosive today because of the pressure on care, care work and care workers (Fraser, 2014; Arruzza et al, 2018). Resistance and collective agency build on the values, ideals and affective relations of the 'non-commodified' zones (Fraser, 2014). It is (mainly) women (of different nationalities, ethnicity, class and migration status), as care workers

Table 3.1: Core dimensions of Fraser's care crisis theory

Dimensions	Indicators
Fundamental dynamic in capitalist societies: contradiction of production and reproduction	Financialised capitalism increasingly obscures the importance of reproductive work for productive work Intensifying commodification and financialisation of care work Social reproduction includes non-commodified zones and values Boundary struggles
Market	Care work increasingly privatised and commodified Recruiting women into the paid workforce Migrant women workers fill the 'care gap' Care work low-paid, low-status
State	Disciplining of states to act in interest of private investors Decreased state investment in social welfare Dual organisation = commodified for those who can pay for it and privatised for those who cannot
Civil society	Role of family and civil society Less time for caring for oneself, families and local society
Gender equality/ feminism	Combination of marketisation and emancipation undermine social protection and define emancipation in market terms, such as 'lean in' feminism, reproduction in contrast to gender equality and giving care work low status

and care-givers, who are at the front of these struggles. It is therefore also a struggle for gender equality, or as Fraser calls it, a struggle for 'parity in participation', which includes recognition, redistribution and representation of care work and care workers (Fraser, 2003, 2008). Moreover, these struggles are boundary struggles, as central to capitalist societies as class struggles are (Fraser, 2016).

Care and social reproduction in the 'women-friendly' Nordic welfare societies

Following this conceptual discussion, in the next sections we contextualise these care crisis dynamics, and show how they have become manifest in the Nordic countries. Women in the Nordic countries have reached a high degree of gender equality with regard to levels of education, labour market participation and democratic agency. In general, welfare state services and social benefits have made it possible for women to combine motherhood, paid work and active citizenship, resulting in women getting a new bargaining position and a higher degree of equality (Borchorst, 1989; Christensen and Siim, 2001). However, the emphasis of paid work in women's liberation did also lead to the reproduction of a male norm regarding which labour counts as work (Holst, 2006; Bjørnholt, 2012) – or, as Fraser might argue, to make unpaid care work and social reproduction invisible as important to societies.

In reality, this is more complex, because paid parental leave and paid sickness leave, as well as regulations on working time, can been seen as recognition of unpaid care work. Fraser points towards the social-democratic welfare state as the ideal model in which transformative policies of redistribution are realised (Fraser, 2003). At the same time, she is critical towards the dual-earner model (Fraser, 1997), which is the basis of the Nordic welfare states. Yet again, we here need to take into consideration the complexities of the Nordic welfare state, as the state acts as additional care-giver providing care service (for example, childcare facilities and elder care) as well as care benefits (such as parental care allowances) (Hansen, 2007).

Central to the Nordic welfare state model is a relatively high degree of decommodification of labour, which means that the individual citizen can exist without having to depend on selling their labour in the market (Esping-Andersen, 1990). Gender researchers add to this an awareness about care work actually being commodified in the Nordic welfare state as it changed (partly) from unpaid work to paid work (Koren, 2012; Aslaksen and Koren, 2014). Dahl and Rasmussen (2012), for instance, argue that elder care in the Nordic welfare states is characterised by both commodification and professionalisation, often partly engineered by the state. Paid care work is (still) mainly organised through the public sector, which means that it is less affected by market forces than in private sector work. At the same time, persistent inequalities mean that gender, ethnicity and class are fundamentally intersecting with paid care work dynamics also in the public sector.

The labour market model is another characteristic of the Nordic societies, with the social partners both alone (the agreement system) and together with the state (the tripartite system) being responsible for most labour market regulation. Trade unions are also, in comparison to the rest of the world, still powerful. This 'Nordic class compromise' (Kjellberg, 1992) balances the unequal power relationship between capital and labour in capitalism, although it does not resolve it, and creates a platform for negotiating contradictory interests (Due et al, 1993). It could be argued that akin to the Nordic class compromise, welfare state and gender equality dynamics have given rise to a form of 'Nordic care compromise'.[1] That is, a balancing of the productive–reproductive contradiction, which does not even out the power relationship, but *moderates* it. Some of the core issues pertaining to care work and reproductive work have been tentatively and temporarily tackled (albeit not resolved) on the basis of concessions and policy mechanisms in parliament, as well as by social partners and a wide range of civil society organisations (CSOs).

Despite the overall similarities in welfare state and labour market models, the Nordic welfare states have significant differences, too. This is clear regarding gender equality arguments, policies and institutions, and in their relationship with care policies and regulation (see Borchorst, 2004). In particular, the levels of institutionalisation of gender equality politics vary, with Sweden at the top and Denmark at the bottom. Traditionally, Norway has stood out with an emphasis on gender difference, and Sweden with a core understanding that society builds on a gender power system. In general, Danish gender equality policies are more liberal and marked by politics of declaration than those in Norway and Sweden. However, structural developments pertaining to financialised capitalism and neoliberalism have led to converging trajectories of these gender equality discourses, for instance with regard to the primacy of gender equality through full-time employment, and to gender equality policies being more liberal. As the profound contradictions of capitalism, as manifested in the fundamental sphere of social reproduction, have become more pronounced and more visible in the Nordic welfare model, it is crucial to understand the crisis dynamics they give rise to.

Care crisis tendencies and resistance in the Nordic welfare societies

Over the last 30 years, New Public Management (NPM) has become the dominant management regime in the public sector, and outsourcing and privatisation of welfare services and public sector work have become common (see, for example, Dahl, 2012). The extent and the level of social security are being scaled back and the disciplining of social security receivers is increasing (Lindberg and Neergaard, 2013). The neoliberal discourse of competitiveness and scarcity permeates policy-making and institutional logics. This, then, brings us back to the starting point of Fraser's systemic critique. In the following, we now draw on the core dimensions and indicators of care crisis that we have summarised in Table 3.1, and discuss how they have become manifest across three central spheres: financialisation, recognition of family and care work, and conflicts and social struggles. The three illustrations from Denmark and Norway highlight specific Nordic variations of care crisis dynamics.

Financialisation of care work in the Nordic welfare state context

The systemic aspects of Fraser's discussion of the contradiction of capital and care require a more differentiated take on neoliberalism and financialisation processes. On a conceptual level, neoliberalism has been much discussed in relation to gender equality, and the welfare state. The linkages between financialisation, or financialised capitalism, and social reproductive work have been less explored. Despite the fact that neoliberalism and financialisation are often used in conjunction, they capture distinct social processes and mechanisms. A useful distinction is provided by Davis and Walsh

(2017: 47): where neoliberalisation can be seen as market-led restructuring, under financialisation 'the means for achieving [this] has a distinctive financial market logic, and thus financial economic paradigm principles have the power to structure neoliberal political-economic objectives'. To understand how this financialised logic affects care and reproductive work in a given institutional and social configuration, there are multiple aspects of financialisation that can be brought into the analysis here.

Financialisation includes a macroeconomic focus on the disciplining of state policies, and hence also welfare state arrangements (for the Swedish case, see Belfrage and Kallifatides, 2018); these are increasingly geared towards the interest of private investors. In the context of care crisis discussions, Farris and Marchetti (2017) capture this aspect by focusing on the 'corporatisation of care'. They distinguish corporatisation from the commodification and marketisation dynamics that are at the core of much research on care dynamics under neoliberal policies and practices. As they explain:

> by corporatization of care ... we refer above all to the growing presence of for-profit companies of various sizes in the provision of care services. Furthermore, the adoption of corporate practices (cost-cutting, business management models, segmentation of the labour process) by public private partnerships and not-for-profit organizations that provide care seems to us to suggest a general reconfiguration of care. (Farris and Marchetti, 2017: 116)

This means a fundamental power shift and reconfiguration of the role of the state vis-a-vis care and reproductive work, as the market becomes 'not simply one of the actors providing care alongside others ... but a key operator whose logic permeates the entire realm of care, causing a complete shift in the functioning and understanding of care provision' (Farris and Marchetti, 2017: 113). In the care and health sector, this results in cutting back on personnel costs by reducing employees' pension rights and relying on a low-paid migrant workforce – often hired on short-term contracts – as well as cutting costs by reducing the quality of care, by, for instance, reducing the frequency of nappy-changes in elderly homes.

We can observe similar dynamics also in the Nordic context across various spheres of social reproduction. In Norway, there has been a rapid expansion of childcare facilities and a concomitant change in formal childcare arrangements for children under the age of three. The expansion of childcare facilities implemented by the red-green coalition government in 2009 was realised predominantly through a large expansion of publicly funded *private* commercial childcare providers. This has led to debates about quality, staffing regulations and concern over childcare companies' high profits and their placing of these profits in tax havens (Lunder and Aastvedt, 2012), as well as the high percentage of subsidies that go to commercial chain businesses compared to smaller childcare facilities (Lunder, 2019). In June 2020, the Norwegian parliament (Storting) passed a new law that further benefited the owners of private childcare companies, removing a previous limitation to 'reasonable profit' and allowing them to freely use their profits (see also Chapter 9 in this volume). At the same time, economic control was moved away from municipalities (through whose budget they are funded) towards the state. With the expansion of commercial childcare providers who shift their profits to tax havens, childcare in Norway is directly coupled to global financialised capitalism.

In Denmark, the relevance of the health industry in overall manufacturing has increased significantly over the last decade (in particular due to pharmaceutical industries, but also thanks to related health technologies). Persistent growth in the export market put the sector share in overall Danish exports at around 16 per cent in 2017 (Dansk Industri, 2018). The financial logic of corporations is increasingly permeating the discourses and policies of relevant areas. As the Danish Industry Confederation put it, this requires a reconfiguration towards 'an innovative domestic market as an exhibition platform for new products and treatments' (Dansk Industri, 2018). This also raises interesting, if broader, questions for the 'crisis of care' discussion; that is the role and potential of technology in resolving, at least temporarily, some of the apparent problems with care provision (see also Chapter 4 in this volume). Solutions to the care crisis are being discussed globally at the level of technological change, and the implementation of these technological solutions is increasing also (maybe even particularly so) in the Nordic welfare states. However, even where broader techno–optimistic perspectives of the future of welfare states are being questioned (for example, Greve, 2017), the discussion does not actually focus on the inherent contradiction between production and social reproduction. Technologies do not alter the fundamental social power relations at the heart of capitalism; rather, more often than not, welfare technologies reinforce disciplining mechanisms and gender inequalities.

Devaluation of care work in families and the misrecognition of mothering

Recognition of social reproduction seems to be particularly difficult within contemporary capitalism; it is, in Fraser's words, viewed as a 'backward residue, an obstacle to advancement that must be sloughed off, one way or another, *en route* to liberation' (Fraser, 2016: 114). Mothers' care is a particularly contentious issue, as it epitomises the image of a 'backward residue', threatening to lure women back to the domestic sphere in contrast to the hard-won right to liberation via paid work. This illustrates Fraser's point that feminism may join forces with market forces.

In contrast to Fraser's US-inspired model, however, in Norway and the other Nordic countries, dual-earner families are supported by a wide 'package' of welfare state benefits. Further, the design of parental leave, with a non-transferable quota for fathers, represents a form of social engineering aimed at redistributing care from mothers to fathers, which is often seen as a realisation of Fraser's 'universal carer' model (1994). On the other hand, the hegemony of the dual-earner model and paid work also implies an implicit devaluation of care, and the efforts to redistribute care to institutions and fathers may have unintended gendered effects in terms of a misrecognition of mothering. The pre-eminence of paid work is reflected in the entitlement to paid parental leave, which is derived from parents' previous paid work, rather than from the infant's need to be cared for by parents. Single mothers are a particularly apt case.

In line with international developments, the retrenchment of economic support and the increasing demands of labour market activation, single parents, predominantly mothers, suffer from a dual shortage of time and money (Roman, 2017a, 2017b). Moreover, the care perspective on lone mothers was replaced by the work and activation perspective in the 1990s (Syltevik, 2015). After a major reduction of the entitlements for single parents in Norway, children of lone parents did significantly worse in school (Reiso, 2014; Løken et al, 2018), illustrating the lasting effects of weakening the mechanisms of social reproduction. The cultural ideal of parenting has shifted towards an almost unilateral support of the dual-earner–dual-carer model. Paid work has become an important element in the construction of the 'good mother', while hands-on caring has become an important part of being a 'good man'. This resonates with the dominant liberal-individualist and gender-egalitarian imaginary of financialised capitalism (Fraser, 2016).

The Norwegian welfare state 'package' for working parents redistributes care to institutions as well as between parents. The paternal quota was first introduced in 1993 as part of a substantial expansion of the total parental leave available to both parents. In contrast, the latest expansions have predominantly redistributed the paid leave by reserving a larger share for fathers, leaving less time available for mothers. While the intention was to redistribute care from mothers to fathers, approximately half of the mothers stay home while the fathers are on paid leave, and one-third of the mothers take additional unpaid leave (Schou, 2019).

The efforts to bring about change by turning men into fathers has also led to changes in gendered status hierarchies and recognition. Fathers' caring has come to represent progress and modernity, while mothers' caring is largely silenced as the backward residue that women should leave behind in order to prioritise paid work, in line with the new ideal of mothers as, first and foremost, workers. The current model also shifts the focus of families from the care and reproductive work that takes place within the family towards prioritising paid work (Bjørnholt, 2012, 2013), thereby eroding social reproduction. Nevertheless, recent developments illustrate the ongoing political struggles over paid work and care in Norway. In 2018, there was an increase in the financial support of parenting – in practice mothering – with rises in the cash-for-care (paid to parents of children aged up to two years who are not in publicly sponsored day-care), in the cash support at birth (for mothers who are not in paid employment), as well as in the universal child allowance. This increase came after 20 years of standstill.

The hegemony of the dual-earner–dual-carer model constitutes a narrow ideal of the appropriate way of life, as parents often struggle to live up to the ideals of double full-time employment and equal sharing of childcare (Bjørnholt and Stefansen, 2018). Studies of families' work and care adaptations, as well as studies of elder care, reveal the inadequacies of institutional care and the costs on families and individual family members in bridging care needs and compensating for deficiencies in the system (Bjørnholt et al, 2017; Dahl, 2017; Bjørnholt and Stefansen, 2018), reflecting gendered patterns of responsibilities. As mothers, women to a larger extent worry about, and take responsibility for, children's well-being in day-care centres (Bjørnholt and Stefansen, 2018). As daughters, women take a larger responsibility and receive less support for ageing parents (Berge et al, 2014). Women were also found to have carried out a much larger share of childcare and household work during the COVID-19 lockdown (Kolberg, 2020).

Women and mothers are caught between the demands of the increasingly strict norms of lifelong, full-time paid work, rising parenting standards, persisting gender inequality in the household and the labour market, and the emotional costs of delegating care to institutions of uneven quality (Bjørnholt and Stefansen, 2018; Bjørnholt, 2019). These conflicting demands are to be met in the context of a misrecognition of care and mothering. The misrecognition of mothering is reflected in the (over-)valuation of paid work, and the implicit devaluation of care (paid and unpaid). It is also reflected in a reduction of support for women's reproductive body work. Examples include the effectivisation of birth and the shortening of time spent in hospitals, and in the reduction of self-responsibilisation and delegation of post-natal care to the family, as well as the negative consequences for mothers' mental health as reflected in post-natal depression rates (Holte and Eberhard-Gran, 2017).

Dynamics of resistance and change in the Danish labour market and beyond

Key to Fraser's care crisis concept is that exploitation and undervaluation of care do not go on without protest. In this section, the consequences of the care crises and the social reproduction struggles these lead to are in focus. Two cases illustrate this: The first case is about conflict, resistance and trade union action among hospital cleaners and housekeepers in hotels. The second is about the conflictual labour market relations in the public sector, starting with wildcat strikes for respect of care work at the bargaining rounds in 2008.[2]

Outsourcing within the service sector has led to heavy pressure on workers' rights and working conditions all over Europe. Clients wish to reduce costs, and the pressure and competition between the many subcontractors have been followed by employers hiring workers who are less protected or to circumventing agreements (Grimshaw et al, 2014; Larsen and Mailand, 2014; Schulten and Buschoff, 2015). Altogether, this has led to an increase in work intensity, with workers complaining about stress and working more hours than they are paid for (Schulten and Buschoff, 2015). This is also the case in the Danish cleaning industry. The outsourcing of hospital cleaning involves a change to less favourable private sector agreements; and in both hospitals and hotels, outsourcing has forced a rise in working speed. Moreover, there is an increase in housekeepers with precarious contracts, often with few guaranteed hours.

Cleaning has always been hard physical work, but the increasing work pressure has left workers with less energy to take care of themselves and others. Moreover, the constant replacement of colleagues (particularly in hotels), limited common language, and little interaction make the building and maintenance of workplace collectives difficult. All in all, affective relations are under pressure, leading to a combination of sadness, apathy and 'escape'. However, we also see a manifestation of anger and a fighting spirit: A group of housekeepers got together and turned to the trade union for support, when a new cleaning system meant that they had to work even faster. The union, together with the employee representatives and spokespersons, formed a group that negotiated with the management, and which, after several months, reached a settlement that partly turned back the changes although not removing the fundamental problems. In addition, protesting both individually and collectively has resulted in some hospitals employing cleaners directly again (see also Hansen, 2019a).

In the public sector NPM, including a wide range of standardisation and control instruments, has led to less autonomy, to feelings of disrespect, and to high numbers of sickness absences (Glerup, 2015; Bilstrup, 2019). However, it has also led to acts of resistance in daily work and to struggles over the ideal of care (Dahl, in Hansen, 2019b). Since the public sector bargaining rounds in 2008, labour relations have been conflictual. The cry for respect for care workers and care work has been persistent, in combination with demands for equal pay. For the bargaining round in 2018, the public sector trade unions changed strategy. They were fed up with the employers using their double role as both employers and legislators to push through with their agenda *and* utilising bargaining rounds to cut down public expenses (Hansen and Mailand, 2019; Høgedahl and Ibsen, 2019). The union leaders, with strong support from members, pledged a musketeer oath on which demands to prioritise and to leave no one behind. Mobilisation happened because of years of reductions in resources and an increasing workload (Høgedahl and Ibsen, 2019) as well as what were seen as provocative actions by the minister in charge of the negotiations (Davali, 2019). The bargaining round ended with a partial victory for the trade unions.

In both cases, the changes following financialisation and neoliberalism have led to conflicts and protest, and negotiations and collective actions have 'pushed' back parts of the changes, but not resolved the care crisis. Important to both collective action and the successful challenge of employer strategies are strong trade unions, as well as labour market regulation and institutions. Institutional and organisational power resources built into the Nordic labour market model constitute some level of protection against financialisation and neoliberalism. Moreover, the protests made visible that financialisation and neoliberalism have not colonialised social reproduction fully, just as Fraser argues (2014). On the contrary, ideals of good care, on how to do your job well, and of solidarity still exist among social reproductive workers and in trade unions. This is also the case among families and their organisations, who supported the workers (in regard to the second case) and took part in public debate and in collective action themselves, for example in the demonstrations 'Hvor er der en voksen?' ((Where is there a grown-up?) organised by parents to children in pre-school care, and initiatives by the CSO Ældresagen (DaneAge Association) (see also Chapter 8 in this volume). In Norway, there have been similar mobilisations against respectively cut downs in day-care and a new model of parental leave (Bjørnholt and Stefansen, 2018). Both ideals *and* organisations and institutions are important to the struggle for a higher status and better material conditions for reproductive work, as well as better care for children, the sick and the elderly. The reproductive struggles show as class conflicts in the labour market, but they do also have a broader dimension as 'boundary struggles', and they include individual citizens and CSOs.

To summarise the key arguments coming out of the illustrations discussed in this section, Table 3.2 provides an overview of the care crisis dynamics in the Nordic welfare states.

Conclusion

In this chapter, we have discussed how Fraser's concept of care crisis can be adopted into the Nordic context. We have operationalised Fraser's thinking into five dimensions, each showing indicators of care crisis, and we have used these to identify care crisis tendencies in the Nordic countries. We can see how indications of a care crisis are both similar and different. We can, for instance, see the manifestation of the individualist and gender-egalitarian

Table 3.2: Summary of care crisis dynamics in Nordic welfare societies

Dimensions	Indicators
Fundamental dynamic in capitalist societies: contradiction of production and reproduction	Increasing financialisation, privatisation and commercialisation of care provision Outsourcing of care work, decreasing social security, and regulation in favour of capital challenge decommodification and embeddedness of the economy Class compromise and care compromise are challenged Yet resistance, struggles and solidarity readiness are widespread and supported by labour market institutions, trade union power and CSOs
Market	Increasing financialisation, privatisation, commodification, corporatisation, and of payment of services and additional 'buying of' better/individualised services Strong discourse of scarcity: 'lack of work force in the future' and restricted economic means. Solution = technological fix
State	Less social democratic welfare state, more 'neoliberal and social investment state', ideology of competitiveness Withdrawal of the state from welfare service provision; more disciplining of and decreasing social benefits Care work regarded an expense and not as contributing to successful business and societal wealth Care workers and trade unions have less influence on care policies and practices Increased focus on management Dual-earner–dual-carer strategy with less involvement from the state
Civil society	More responsibility placed on families Caring for oneself and for communities are overshadowed by obligation to participate in labour market and on self-support More vulnerability, weakened communities
Gender equality/feminism	Gender equality = sameness and full-time paid employment Increasing focus on fathering and men's gender equality Mothering and unpaid care work have less status

discourses Fraser points to in financialised capitalism in the Nordic welfare state; however, practices and institutional arrangements of the care compromise are (still) prevalent. Yet, the fall in welfare services, de-skilling of professional care work, low pay, outsourcing, bad working conditions, pressure on workers' rights, and less influence, all challenge both the care- and the class–compromise. Efforts to change the gendered division of care in the family dovetail with the two–earner model and perpetuate the reallocation of time from care to paid work, fitting all too well into a neoliberal frame. Further, the effort to validate and promote fathers' caring in this context may also lead to a devaluation and misrecognition of mothers and other groups' caring, following and deepening gendered, classed and ethnic divides.

The reproduction of a male norm on work following the emphasis on paid work for obtaining gender equality has increased and shows as a specific variant of the Nordic care crisis putting even more pressure on unpaid care work. Yet, the cases also show other Nordic variations on the care crisis: how taxes support private business, not as direct industrial subsidies, but through outsourcing of welfare services; how in the US, a call for mothers' responsibility for care is reproducing gendered inequalities, while the invisibility of love and care work in families and the importance of mothering in the Nordic context is reproducing gendered inequalities; and how labour market institutions and organisations, in combination with strong CSOs and a general 'solidarity readiness' (Caraker, 2017), render resistance to neoliberalism and financialisation possible.

The discussion of concrete crisis dynamics of financialised capitalism in the Nordic welfare state also raises crucial issues relevant to thinking about political crisis, including the possibilities for alternatives, resistance and social struggles. Nordic institutions and organisations, as well as ideals about care and solidarity, render resistance possible, and mitigate the consequences of neoliberalism and financialisation. It remains to be seen, though, whether more transformative changes will occur; either in the direction of deep structural change to a more sustainable model as in Fraser's outlook, or in other ways, in which societies could be organised around care in line with Tronto's *homines curans*, also in the Nordics.

Since the welfare state and the collective agreement system are so important in regulating and mitigating the consequences of market activities, since welfare services and social security have been important to gender equality, *and* since public sector care work is the major workplace for women, changes within this system (for example, cutting down on services and social security as well as deteriorating working conditions) affect gender equality negatively, challenging both the class compromise and the care compromise, and rendering the Nordic societies less sustainable. In conclusion, Fraser's framework, as we have shown, can indeed provide a fruitful tool for analysing how the crisis of care is manifesting in the Nordic welfare states, but only if it is contextualised with a historically, institutionally and culturally specific analysis.

Note

[1] The notion of a care compromise as a counterpart to the much better known class compromise has developed from a workshop discussion in the Nordic Care Crisis Network. Hansen, Bjørnholt and Horn have subsequently refined and defined it.

[2] The case about commercial cleaning builds on data and analyses from a research project about worker solidarity in the Danish labour market conducted by Lise Lotte Hansen and funded by the Danish Research Council for Society and

54

Business. The case about conflicts in the public sector builds mainly on Dahl (2017), Davali (2019), Høgedahl (2019) and Hansen and Mailand (2019).

References

Arruzza, C., Bhattacharya, T. and Fraser, N. (2018) 'Notes for a feminist manifesto', *New Left Review*, 114(Nov/Dec): 113–134.

Aslaksen, J. and Koren, C. (2014) 'Reflections on unpaid household work, economic growth, and consumption possibilities' in M. Bjørnholt and A. McKay (eds) *Counting on Marilyn Waring: New Advances in Feminist Economics*, Bradford: Demeter Press, pp 57–71.

Belfrage, C. and Kallifatides, M. (2018) Financialisation and the new Swedish model. *Cambridge Journal of Economics*, 42(4): 875–899.

Berge, T., Øien, H. and Jacobsen, L.N. (2014) *Formell og uformell omsorg. Samspill mellom familien og velferdsstaten, NOVA paperseries 3/2014*, Oslo: Norwegian Social Research.

Bhattacharya, T. (2017) *Social Reproduction Theoy: Remapping Class, Recentering Oppression*, London: Pluto.

Bilstrup, M. (2019) 'Styringen af de offentlige ansatte har taget overhånd', *Debatindlæg Tidsskrift for Arbejdsliv*, 21(2): 100–103.

Bjørnholt, M. (2012) 'From work-sharing couples to equal parents: Changing perspectives of men and gender equality' in M.J. Samuelsson, C. Krekula and M. Åberg (eds) *Gender and Change: Power, Politics and Everyday Practices*, Karlstad: Karlstad University Press, pp 53–72.

Bjørnholt, M. (2013) 'The vulnerability approach: A way of bridging the equality-difference dilemma?', *Retfærd*, 36(3): 25–44.

Bjørnholt, M. (2018) 'How to make what really matters count in economic decision-making: Care, domestic violence, gender responsive budgeting, macro-economic policies and human rights' in V. Gorgino and Z.D. Walsh (eds) *Co-Designing Economics in Transition: Radical Approaches in Dialogue with Contemplative Social Sciences*, London: Palgrave Macmillan, pp 135–159.

Bjørnholt, M. (2019) 'Mothering and the economy' in L. O'Brien, A. Hallstein, M. O'Reilly and G. Vandenbeld (eds) *The Routledge Companion to Motherhood*, London and New York: Routledge, pp 389–401.

Bjørnholt, M. and McKay, A. (eds) (2014) *Counting on Marilyn Waring: New Advances in Feminist Economics*, Bradford: Demeter Press.

Bjørnholt, M. and Stefansen, K. (2018) 'Same but different: Polish and Norwegian parents' work–family adaptations in Norway', *Journal of European Social Policy*, 29(2): 292–304.

Bjørnholt, M., Stefansen, K., Gashi, L. and Seeberg, M.L. (2017) 'Balancing acts: Policy frameworks and family care strategies in Norway' in T. Sirovátka and J. Válková (eds) *Understanding Care Policies in Changing Times: Experiences and Lessons from the Czech Republic and Norway*, Masaryk: Centre for Studies of Democracy and Culture, pp 161–184.

Borchorst, A. (1989) 'Kvinderne, velfærdsstaten og omsorgsarbejdet', *Politica*, 21(2): 132–148.

Borchorst, A. (2004) 'Skandinavisk ligestillingspolitik tur-retur, på dansk billet', *Nytt Norsk Tidsskrift*, 21(3–4): 264–274.

Borchorst, A. and Siim, B. (2010) 'The women-friendly welfare states revisited', *NORA – Nordic Journal of Feminist and Gender Research*, 10(2): 90–98.

Brenner, N., Peck, J. and Theodore, N. (2010) 'Variegated neoliberalization: Geographies, modalities, pathways', *Global Networks*, 10(2): 182–222.

Caraker, E. (2017) *Fællesskab gør forskel. En APL III-forskningsrapport om lønmodtagerinteresser og værdier belyst ud fra interviews*, København: FTF/LO.

Christensen, A.-D. and Siim, B. (2001) *Køn, demokrati og modernitet: mod nye politiske identiteter*, Copenhagen: Hans Reitzels Forlag.

Dahl, H.M. (2012) 'Neo-liberalism meets the Nordic welfare state: Gaps and silences', *NORA – Nordic Journal of Feminist and Gender Research*, 20(4): 283–288.

Dahl, H.M. (2017) *Struggles in (Elderly) Care: A Feminist View*, London: Palgrave Macmillan.

Dahl, H.M. and Rasmussen, B. (2012) 'Paradoxes of elder care: The Nordic model' in A. Kamp and H. Hviid (eds) *Elder care in Transition: Management, Meaning and Identity at Work. A Scandinavian Perspective*, Copenhagen: Copenhagen Business School Press, pp 29–49.

Dalla Costa, M. and James, S. (1975) *The Power of Women and the Subversion of the Community*, Bristol: Falling Wall Press.

Dansk Industri (2018) 'Ti års fremgang for sundhedsindustrien', *Dansk Industri*, Available from: https://www.danskindustri.dk/arkiv/analyser/2018/9/ti-ars-fremgang-for-sundhedsindustrien/ [accessed 24 November 2020].

Davali, Y. (2019) *Solidaritet på tværs af faggrupper – en analyse af arbejdstagersolidaritet under OK18*, Speciale i Socialvidenskab, Roskilde: Roskilde Universitet.

Davis, A. and Walsh, C. (2017) 'Distinguishing financialization from neoliberalism', *Theory, Culture and Society*, 34(5–6): 27–51.

Dowling, E. (2017) 'In the wake of austerity: Social impact bonds and the financialisation of the welfare state in Britain', *New Political Economy*, 22(3): 294–310.

Due, J., Madsen, J.S. and Jensen, C.S. (1993) *Den danske Model. En historisk sociologisk analyse af det kollektive aftalesystem*, Copenhagen: Jurist- og Økonomforbundets Forlag.

Esping-Andersen, G. (1990) *The Three Worlds of Welfare Capitalism*, New York: Princeton University Press.

Farris, S. and Marchetti, S. (2017) 'From the commodification to the corporatization of care: European perspectives and debates', *Social Politics*, 24(2): 109–131.

Ferber, M.A. and Nelson, J.A. (eds) (1993) *Beyond Economic Man: Feminist Theory and Economics*, Chicago and London: University of Chicago Press.

Folbre, N. (2001) *The Invisible Heart Economics and Family Values*, New York: The New Press.

Fraser, N. (1997) *Justice Interruptus*, New York and London: Routledge.

Fraser, N. (2003) 'Social justice in the age of identity politics' in N. Fraser and A. Honneth (eds) *Redistribution and Recognition?* London and New York: Verso, pp 7–109.

Fraser, N. (2008) *Scales of Justice: Reimagining Political Space in a Globalizing World*, Cambridge: Polity Press.

Fraser, N. (2009) 'Feminism, capitalism and the cunning of history', *New Left Review*, 56(March/April): 117.

Fraser, N. (2013) 'A triple movement? Parsing the politics of crisis after Polanyi', *New Left Review*, 81(May/June): 119–132.

Fraser, N. (2014) 'Behind Marx's hidden abode: For an expanded conception of capitalism', *New Left Review*, 86 (March/April): 55–72.

Fraser, N. (2016) 'Contradictions of capital and care', *New Left Review*, 100(July/August): 99–117.

Glerup, J. (ed) (2015) *Bladet fra munden – mod og vilje til et godt arbejdsliv*, Copenhagen: Dansk Sygeplejeråd.

Greve, B. (2017) *Technology and the Future of Work: The Impact on Labour Markets and Welfare States*, Cheltenham: Edward Elgar.

Grimshaw, D., Cartwright, J., Keizer, A., Rubery, J., Hadjivassiliou, K. and Rickard C. (2014) *Coming Clean: Contractual and Procurement Practices*, Institute for Employment Studies, Equality and Human Rights Commission, Research report 96.

Hansen, L.L. (2007) 'From flexicurity to flexicarity? Gendered perspectives on the Danish model', *Journal of Social Sciences*, 3(2): 88–93.

Hansen, L.L. (2019a) 'Ligestilling eller "a no-life-life"? Rengøringsarbejde, social dumping og retfærdighed' in L.L. Hansen (ed) *Køn, magt & mangfoldighed*, Frydenlund: Frydenlund Academic, pp 196–218.

Hansen, L.L. (ed) (2019b) *Køn, magt & mangfoldighed*, Frydenlund: Frydenlund Academic.

Hansen, N.W. and Mailand, M. (2019) 'OK18- en forklaring af forløbet og en ny forståelse af magtbalancen', *Tidsskrift for Arbejdsliv*, 21(2): 10–27.

Henderson, H. (1996) *Building a Win-Win World: Life Beyond Global Economic Warfare*, San Francisco: Berrett-Koehler.

Hernes, H.M. (1987) *Welfare State and Woman Power: Essays in State Feminism*, Oslo: Scandinavian University Press.

Hochschild, A.R. (1995) 'The culture of politics: Traditional, postmodern, cold-modern, and warm-modern ideals of care', *Social Politics: International Studies in Gender, State & Society*, 2(3): 331–346.

Høgedahl, L. (2019) *Den danske model i den offentlige sektor. Danmark i et nordisk perspektiv*, Copenhagen: DJØF Forlag.

Høgedahl, L. and Ibsen, F. (2019) 'OK18: Solidaritetspagt, musketeer-ed, massemobilisering og tæt på konflikt i den offentlige sektor', *Tidsskrift for Arbejdsliv*, 21(2): 47–66.

Holst, C. (2006) 'Statsfeminismen og nasjonalstaten', *Kvinder, Køn & Forskning*, 15(4): 5–16.

Holte, A. and Eberhard-Gran, M. (2017) 'Fødselsdepresjon. Fy skam til Regjeringen. Aftenposten', Available from: https://www.aftenposten.no/meninger/debatt/i/7a07o/Fodselsdepresjon-Fy-skam-til-Regjeringen--Arne-Holte-og-Malin-Eberhard-Gran [accessed 24 November 2020].

Kittay, E.F. (1999) *Love's Labor: Essays on Women, Equality and Dependency*, New York and London: Routledge.

Kjellberg, A. (1992) 'Sweden: Can the model survive' in A. Ferner and R. Hyman (eds) *Industrial Relations in the New Europe*, Oxford: Blackwell, pp 88–142.

Kolberg, L. (2020) *Likestilling i Korona-tider – hvem gjør hva?* Rapport 2/2020, Hamar: Likestillingssenteret.

Koren, C. (2012) *Kvinnenes rolle i norsk økonomi*, Oslo: Universitetsforlaget.

Larsen, T.P. and Mailand, M. (2014) *Bargaining for Social Rights in Sectors (BARSORIS) – National Report Denmark*, FAOS rapport 142, København.

Lindberg, I. and Neergaard, A. (2013) 'Mellan Marx och Polanyi: Ett nytt landskap för kollektivt handlande och facklig förnyelse' in I. Lindberg and A. Neergaard (eds) *Bortom Horisonten. Fackets vägval i globaliseringens tid*, Stockholm: Premiss Förlag, pp 13–38.

Luøken, K.V., Lommerud, K.E. and Reiso, K.H. (2018) 'Single mothers and their children: Evaluating a work-encouraging welfare reform', *Journal of Public Economics*, 167(Nov): 1–20.

Lunder, T.E. (2019) *Finansiering av private barnehager Vurderinger av foreslåtte endringer i tilskuddsmodellen*, Bø: Telemarksforskning.

Lunder, T.E. and Aastvedt, A. (2012) *Kostnader i barnehager i 2011 og nasjonale satser for 2013*, Bø: Telemarksforsking.

Mies, M. (1986) *Patriarchy and Accumulation on a World Scale: Women in the International Division of Labour*, London and New York: Zed Books.

O'Hara, S. (2014) 'Everything needs care: Toward a relevant contextual view of the economy' in M. Bjørnholt and A. McKay (eds) *Counting on Marilyn Waring: New Advances in Feminist Economics*, Bradford: Demeter Press, pp 37–55.

Reiso, K. (2014) *Young Unemployed, Single Mothers and Their Children*, Phd dissertation, University of Bergen.

Roman, C. (2017a) 'Lone mothers with low income face obstacles to practice their mothering', *Sociologisk forskning*, 54(4): 303–306.

Roman, C. (2017b) 'Between money and love: Work–family conflict among Swedish low-income single mothers', *Nordic Journal of Working Life Studies*, 7(3): 23–41.

Schou, L. (2019) *Fornuft og følelser – En studie av mors og fars uttak av foreldrepenger*, Rapport 2/2019, Oslo: Arbeids- og velferdsdirektoratet.

Schulten, T. and Buschoff, K.S. (2015) *Sector-Level Strategies Against Precarious Employment in Germany: Evidence from Construction, Commercial Cleaning, Hospitals and Temporary Agency Work*, WSI Diskussionspapier 197, Düsseldorf: Hans Böckler Stiftung.

Syltevik, L.J. (2015) 'Paid and unpaid work in the Norwegian welfare state: The case of the lone mother allowance', *Annals of the University of Bucharest, Political Science Series*, 17(1): 5–18.

Tronto, J.C. (1993) *Moral Boundaries: A Political Argument for an Ethic of Care*, New York and London: Routledge.

Tronto, J.C. (2013) *Caring Democracy: Markets, Equality, and Justice*, New York and London: New York University Press.

Tronto, J. (2017) 'There is an alternative: Homines curans and the limits of neoliberalism', *International Journal of Care and Caring*, 1(1): 27–43.

Wærness, K. (1978) 'The invisible welfare state: Women's work at home', *Acta Sociologica*, 21(1_suppl): 193–207.

Wærness, K. (1984) 'The rationality of caring', *Economic and Industrial Democracy*, 5(2): 185–211.

Waring, M. (1988) *If Women Counted: Towards a Feminist Economics*, San Francisco: Harper & Row.

4

Crisis of care: a problem of economisation, of technologisation or of politics of care?

Anne Kovalainen

Introduction

The question of care, and how to organise it, is globally pertinent and touches not only gendered care and dependencies, but also ethics of care, reflected in the ways in which care is governed and what becomes emphasised in the analyses. Societal discourses on the governance of care revolve around the issues of quality (ethics), costs (economy) and remedies (technology). The three discourses hold separate realms in research but enmesh in everyday life, visible for example in the reactions, actions and repercussions in the current COVID-19 pandemic. Globally, the COVID-19 crisis societal discourses seem to constitute three differing logics: the costs to economies due to lockdowns and restrictions; the costs to citizens' health and lives due to loosening restrictions; and the restoration of 'normality' by vaccination as remedy. Ethics cut through these discourses by questioning, for example, the values in the political decisions and the politically set national priorities and reactions.

Seeing care as an 'informal' or 'formal', or 'market' or 'non-market' activity aligns with other societal contracts and arrangements that are part of societally accepted patterns, cultures, policies and gendered social contracts (Kovalainen, 2004), but also vehicles for transferring embedded discriminatory and/or unequal practices and processes. With the emergence of market governance mechanisms, the categories of 'public' and 'private', and formal and informal, are blurred and fluid. The bending of boundaries in the organisational and institutional arrangements is reality (for example Kovalainen and Sundin, 2012; Sandberg and Elliott, 2019). The creation of quasi-markets (for example Le Grand and Bartlett, 1993) intensified 'marketisation', that is, the adoption of market as a governance form in the public sphere. This 'market making' is just one example of the processes of economisation. 'Economisation' refers to the economic instrumental rationalities, processes and practices that increasingly rule social life – and even research (for example Çalışkan and Callon, 2009; Fraser, 2014; Vogel, 2018; Wenzlaff, 2019). 'Financialisation' for its part follows economisation and banks on capital formation: in care, it can range from global investment funds acquiring private care homes (Horton, 2017) to the attempts to standardise care as private equity and transform care into a tradable asset.[1] In this process, technologies align with financialisation.

Globally pertinent questions regarding the organising of care address not only contents, ethics and policies, but also costs and deficits. In the Global North, migrant women have supplemented the void of care (Parreñas, 2001; Yeates, 2009; Anderson and Shutes, 2014), for example. But when the cost – and not lack of – care workers is the main rationale in global care migration, the costs, politics and the ethics of care arrangements transcend national boundaries.

The stated societal 'care crises' consist of complex moral, political, economic and social dimensions, which need to be contextualised, with the limits of validity articulated, clarity in the definitions and frames used, and delimitations of the analyses laid out. The 'care crisis' does not have one, but many definitions, with analyses that are embedded and rooted in several disciplinary fields, with epistemic differences and delineations. Thus, the care crisis becomes differently understood and interpreted, and the lenses used in the analyses are multiple.

This chapter addresses the disconnectedness of the societal, economic and political aspects of care in the academic literature. The chapter asks why the academic discussions on care, rather than addressing the entangled, complex and enmeshed care, operate through separate and disconnected fields and lenses.

Several types of academic literature are drawn upon in this chapter, such as feminist scholarship within the field of the ethics of care (Held, 2006; Tronto, 2010; Williams, 2011; Collins, 2015), economics (Çalışkan and Callon, 2009; Wenzlaff, 2019), science and technology studies (Wilson, 2002; Schillmeier and Doménech, 2016), and critical studies on technology (for example Pols and Moser, 2009).

The chapter concludes that the offered remedies for the crisis of care are mainly technological and techno-material in nature, and based on digitalisation, technological efficiency, surveillance and AI-based algorithmic solutions, while the remedies that relate to the *politics of care* are left untouched in these technological discourses, practices and realities. This chapter proposes that the crisis of care should be analysed contextually as a process. Technologies of care are partially a governance solution of the economisation of the crisis of care and because of that they need to be addressed mainly as part of the *political* problem, and not solely as a technological solution.

Modes of care crisis present in research

This chapter addresses three fields of care research, 'ethics of care', 'technologies of care' and 'economics of care', to find out if crossing over of disconnectedness with elements of boundary work, such as epistemological transactions between fields, takes place.

One key aspect in the stated crisis is structural, which follows the nationally constituted economic and political solutions in the welfare policies (Fraser, 2013, 2016; Levitsky, 2014). The liberalisation of organising principles of the welfare services in European and Nordic countries – creation of quasi-markets, purchaser–provider split, decreasing state provision and increased privatisation of services (Le Grand, 1984; Daly and Lewis, 1998; Kovalainen, 1999) – provided ground for commodification of care work and further invasion of market logics into all activities, the public sector included. Markets do not, however, supply a normative foundation for care organising; as Krippner (2005, 2011) notes, the market is a mechanism for functions, not a principle of justice.

For rather a long time, the ethics of care research did not incorporate commodification or economisation into the analyses of care, or into the embodied and situated care ethics, but instead addressed the higher grounds, the moral value of care. But care is commodified. Hospitals as buildings and brands, and care business models are already part of the equity markets and tradable capital in asset management. Financial capitalism as a concept means that financial markets have a growing influence and equity formation has an impact on not only the economy, but on society. Financialisation thus not only affects institutions, but also everyday lives and non-economic spheres of society (for example Aglietta and Breton, 2001; Krippner, 2011; Levitsky, 2014). Technology as a remedy to the care crisis is fuelled by financialisation, but care as an embodied work turns into a financial asset only if its commodification leads to capital gains. In the wake of the care crisis, the questions of who does care work, and who pays for it, emerge intertwined with gender, but also with money, public–private divisions and inequalities of new kinds that are built into the current health care and welfare systems.

For the purposes of this chapter, it is important to dissect how care crises are acknowledged as 'crises' in research. More generally, what types of discursive spaces exist and how do the socio–material crises become constructed, and consequently, what possible remedies are recognised? Even if care crisis is a broad and malleable concept with a wide range of meanings, three different types of discussions are addressed here. The interest is to recognise the possible boundary work between the different discussions, and the role of technology as the legitimating vehicle for care-related political solutions.

Care crisis as an articulated moral question

The formation of the 'care space' in the welfare state and social philosophy literature is well researched and analysed by prominent feminist sociologists, political scientists and philosophers addressing the question of care in differing ways in relation to welfare state formation, changes and political state questions (for example Lewis; Williams; Daly; Lister; Tronto; Fraser; see also Chapter 2 in this volume).[2] The addressing of the care crisis relates not only to the care processes, dependencies and vulnerabilities in care relations, but also to the transformations in the role of the state. Yeatman (2018) has pointed to the reorganisation of state power in forms that are less open for feminist challenge, for example. Developments of the welfare state and blurring boundaries of organisations are examples of that.

The question of 'to whom care belongs' is conceptually close to the questions of classical moral theory (Held, 2006), and partly contrasting with the idea of 'feminine' voices and moral principles of care (Gilligan, 1987). Held developed the ethics of care towards a general moral theory relevant not only to the so-called private realms, but also to medical practices (Held, 2006). The care experienced and care received as bodily engagement transits these principles into intersectionalities and lived practices (for example Hamington, 2015). The ethics of care relates to the moral definitions of the care crisis more generally, as care ethics relates to the arrangements of care and deficiencies in them (for example Sevenhuijsen, 2004). The prescriptive ethics of care focuses on the professional caring relationships, and thus brings forward normative definitions of good care (Menon, 2018). The policy documents act as 'vehicles for normative paradigms' (Sevenhuijsen, 2004: 14–15) that configure knowledge in ways that certain positions become privileged and others not, for example.

How does the moral dimension of the care crisis relate to the aspects in ethics of care? For Tronto (1995), the moral disposition and a set of moral sensibilities, issues and practices arise from taking care as a central aspect of human existence. Tronto (for example 2010) and earlier, Sevenhuijsen et al (2003), view care as a continuous social process characterised by a holistic view of care not restricted to and concerning only privatised relations, but more importantly, social and political institutions as well as societal values. The ethics of care is for them one measuring stick for the normative frameworks of social and political value systems of the state.

The question of the crisis is also dependent on the aspects of normatively defined 'good' and solutions distilled through that definition. According to Pols (2015), care ethicists see it as their task to define or normatively describe the essence of good care, but it may create a problem from the political point of view (see, for example, Walker, 2007). What happens to the normatively described essence of good care if the parameters for or practices of care change? This may happen with the introduction of technology, as the description of the essence of good care may be subject to change.

In empirical studies concerning the elements of 'good care', technology within care – as devices or assisting tools, or as replacements for humans – is usually not ranked high as an element of good care by care professionals (for example Nieboer et al, 2014). Similarly, among care professionals, technology is not considered as the best solution for the deficiencies in care. A typical research result among care professionals is that technology is seldom seen as a replacement for humans in any adequate meaning, despite the visions of robots that abound (Pols, 2012, 2015; Coeckelbergh, 2015). Several empirical studies have shown that care professionals appreciate the technology they already use in care if professional values, tailoring of technology and training for the users are present both in the design and in the use of technology (for example Palm, 2013). Usability challenges with technologies continue to have and have had unintended consequences, ranging from patient harm due to poor electronic patient registries (Ratwani et al, 2019) to biased gender testing of technology (Schiebinger and Schraudner, 2011).

One conclusion from the literature is that the ethics of care literature and technological care literature do not align with the scrutinised care. The ethics and ideals of good care do not necessarily go hand in hand with technology (Walker, 2007; Nieboer et al, 2014; Timmerman et al, 2019). Technologies may offer new care practices and improvements, and in doing so, they transform the understandings of what good care is about. The possibility for tensions and conflicts in values needs articulation, however, as the construction of principles and values are realised in the multitude of practices of care, and in those processes, the technology should align to *serve and support* values *in* care, not set the value standards *for* care.

Care crisis as an articulated economic question

When the crisis of care is articulated and framed in monetary terms in research, it is typically addressed as *'spending'*, *'expense'*, *'cost'* or *'projections of expenditure'*, such as budgets. The monetary measures of care are deceptive, however, as they conflate many of the unmeasurable elements of care and persuade with the 'clarity' of numbers. For example, the rising costs of health and care are estimated, for example by the OECD (2019a, 2019b). In these estimates, the health and care expenditure costs are calculated as a share of gross dmoestic product (GDP). The GDP as conventionally defined differs from welfare; for example, it does not include the non–market activities that bear on economic well-being (for example Dynan and Sheiner, 2018). While mainstream cost projections concentrate on monetary values and how care is financed, there are fewer projections concerning the quality of care, accessibility to care, affordability and availability of care in relation to costs, or in relation to informal unpaid care. The growth of requests for broader measures of welfare which are not bound to GDP is evident (for example Jorgenson, 2010). While many of these discourses are pertinent, they also raise new questions regarding the relationship between economy, values and care practices.

The crisis of care as an *economic* question corresponds to the lack of funds within the health and care sector, and/or the lack of funds of those in need of care. It is a well-known fact that many high-income countries have cut public health-care spending since the global economic downturn and austerity since 2008. The economic crisis, manifested by job and wealth losses and financial fragility, leads to reductions in the use of routine medical care, and the cross-national differences are aligned with differences in the out-of-pocket costs of care across countries (WHO, 2014; Lusardi et al, 2015). The economic crisis of care is highly value-laden, and structural.

Even if the boundaries between 'public and non-profit' and 'private and for-profit' activities may seem clear, when based on the universality of care, payment for care, insurance policies and out-of-pocket cash payments, there are many more dynamic transactions and blurring of the boundaries in the actual functions, organising, practices of operating and activity logics of arranging care. The adoption of market mechanisms as one integral mechanism in the public sector has brought marketisation into public activities and changed the ways in which care is organised, delivered and monitored within the public sector. It is one manifestation of the New Public Management (Kovalainen and Sundin, 2012), but more importantly, it is not limited to financial or economic transactions. The bidding and procurement systems in public provision and purchasing emphasise and underline the economies of care. The cost-cutting mechanisms in the form of quasi-market ideology permeate both the public and the private sector, from health and social care, cleaning work to library service work.

The transformation of the Nordic welfare model – even if it has not changed its basic principles of universality and publicly funded and at least partially publicly provided care – means that many of the private sector practices and organising models are in use in the public sector care regime. Managerial practices and processes, the organising of work, responsibilities and even job titles resemble one another. The awareness of the costs increased with the economic crisis of the 1990s in some countries (such as the UK, Finland) and finance became part of the everyday vocabulary (Simonen and Kovalainen, 1998; Kovalainen and Österberg-Högstedt, 2011; Wouters and McKee, 2017). Indeed, this 'monetary care' was adopted as one new task among the old tasks in care jobs, first because of budget cuts, and then through budget responsibilities, in the 1990s, and almost equally in both the public and private sectors. 'Monetary and budget issues' are one key part of the new responsibilities in all care jobs aligned with the economic crisis, the growth of entrepreneurialism and the rise of New Public Management. The transformation and restructuring of welfare services concerned the gendered care work. The active role of the public sector in creating and constructing markets, and shaping the existing markets, meant the immersion of New Public Management ideology into social and health care sector work practices, and for many women, doing the 'worrying' about the finances of care in their everyday care work, ideological displacement from care ethics to monetary ethics.

Research suggests that in order to maintain their legitimacy, care organisations and care corporations engage in two different operational logics (French and Miller, 2012). These logics for their part increasingly engage all care activities, processes and practices with either *technological innovations* or *entrepreneurial activities*, irrespective of whether the production logic of care is public or private. These engagements of technologies and entrepreneurialism are at the core of the new politics of care both in the public sector and in the private sector. It is highly interesting that only the technological innovations, to be implemented within the existing organisations, but not entrepreneurial activities offering new organisational models, are being offered by politics as solutions to economic crises.

Empirical studies on the economies of care at the population level show a global rise in the number of countries that allow people to access their health data electronically, but fewer than half of them have the digital tools available for it (OECD, 2019b). The emphasis on the economies of care has increased the grey economy and labours of love by relatives: if care services, such as transportation for disabled persons, are not available in sparsely populated areas, technologies can be a helpful solution, but only to a certain point. The ministerial and official reports seldom tackle the new social questions in relation to the cost savings that new technology solutions bring. Economies of care should not detach values from that equation.

Care crisis as an articulated techno-political question

In political discourses, the care crisis refers often to a structural mismatch between the needs of care and inputs to care, or to the unsustainable organising of care systems and commodification of care through profit-making institutional solutions. Partly because of this, the crisis of care is articulated through a variety of discourses: the increasing care needs of the growing elderly population, the care deficits borne from the declining number of care jobs and expenditure due to state budget cuts, to mention a few. These structural aspects govern much of the rising inequalities within the care systems and the rising price tags of the care, and put the political system into the limelight.

Policies and practices also reach care practices and processes diffusely, in contrast to articulated or formal care and health policies. Work practices, new technologies adopted in care processes, and decisions to use AI or apps in care-related work are all examples of the ways in which technologies become amalgamated into care, without deliberate policies, or articulated and written policies or decisions. *Techno-politics*, a mode of politics based on techno-scientific knowledge that informs decision-making activities, functions as an organising principle in care practices (for example Sampedro, 2011; Saborowski and Kollak, 2015). How do techno-politics change care governance and/or practices? Technologies are incorporated into all work, care work included. Solutions such as AI, algorithms, apps and robotics are rendered with care and aligned with care work practices and processes. The technological processes in care often take place either under 'cost-cutting' or 'development' procedures, such as work procedure and control apps, or monitoring devices.

Part of the care work is subsumed with innovations and AI-operating robots and ICT-dependent care devices and supporting, controlling or surveillance mechanisms. Surveillance is regulated through privacy laws, such as the General Data Protection Regulation (GDPR) in Europe, with attempts to lessen the opaqueness of surveillance. No such legislation exists in the US at the federal level (Ajunwa, 2017). Monitoring work performance through timetables is part of the new work practices of digitalisation. The new practices become adopted through gradual work practice adoption and through cultures of experimentation: in a nationwide survey in 2019, half of the nurses in Spain used health apps for professional purposes, even without validation of the apps by the health or professional institutions, and similar results were found in a UK study (Mayer et al, 2019). One of the interesting questions for further analysis is how financialisation, technologies and state interests align in care practices, and to what extent technologies transform the different elements of care.

Technologies offer novelty aspects to care work, and they provide care workers as users with tech prowess and turn them into active agents, developers and co-creators of care technologies. It is through the practices in actual care work where the use, intensification and entanglement of technology in every aspect of care takes place. In this process, the New Public Management governance undoubtedly enables the enactments of technologies in care work and in care practices to become part of the entrepreneurial solution to the problem at hand. Technologies offer solutions to care work and care activities, and during the global COVID-19 crisis, telemedicine and virtual software platforms, chatbots and wearable devices are being adopted as part of the new care routines. Technologies are powerful agents in reshaping care and redefining the view into the care crisis.

Techno-politics in care come with a number of ethical, social, political and legal challenges, including changes and redefinitions in care work cultures, ranges of expertise and subjects of care.

Technology as a remedy?

Technology as a techno-political or socio-technical 'remedy' to the care crisis relates to the novelty of the technological solutions offered. The use of telehealth technologies in home care (home telehealth) has seen globally a rapid growth since the late 1990s (Demiris, 2016). Most often, the offered technological remedies are based on successful and widely used health monitoring cases, where wideband connections and mobile phone apps are used to monitor patients in their homes, often without patient interference or participating activity, such as remote monitoring of pacemakers, and blood pressure and glucose monitors which require only minimal activity from the patient. Pacemaker remote monitoring requires a broadband connection, allowing the monitoring to take place hundreds of miles away without the patient participating in the monitoring work. The data surveillance informs of deviations, and a human expert interferes with a physical check-up only if the data alerts the need to interfere. COVID-19 is acting as a rapid catalyst for the growth of digital care services ranging from mental health interventions and delivering teletherapy to more somatic consultations, with the need to meet systems- and policy-level requirements (Taylor et al, 2020).

The technological care practices have produced positive outcomes in terms of health monitoring (Hampton, 2012), assistance in mobility and care work (for example Beedholm et al, 2016) accuracy of the data and also in terms of cost reduction (for example Bedaf et al, 2015), just to mention a few examples. This list could be extended ad infinitum, with global (IBM Watson, Google Health), national and even local or consumer-targeted variations in health and care trials, uses and technological adaptations. These examples bring forward the technology as part of the care procedure and augmentation, and all these examples mentioned also require well-developed – and universally available – health and technology infrastructures, in order to function properly.

One of the discourses in the health-care robotics literature is that the digitalisation of care, that is, the technology-assisted care devices and monitoring of care, reduces the monetary expenses and costs of care. Howeever, the connection between care technologies and cost structures is not straightforward. The historical analyses of the cost growth in health care show that especially in the US, but also elsewhere, the private insurance system has been a major factor in the growth of health care costs and the major promoter in the development of new medical technologies (Peden and Freeland, 1995; Chernew et al, 1998; Bodenheimer, 2005). Technologies may, when adopted, directly lower the costs, as for example the remote-controlled surveillance system diminishes the number of in-person patient visits at their homes and thus also personnel costs. However, the indirect costs of remote care may also be much higher and, overall, more difficult to calculate. Functioning technologies in care presuppose robust societal and legal infrastructures, IT infrastructure included, as well as training of health-care personnel and modifications to workflows and information flows in health and social care infrastructure. Most technological health-care innovations will generate higher expenditure on health-care services at the aggregate level, but also contradictory evidence exists: a body of evidence indicates that the cost of technology varies by disease and that, overall, technology lowers the care costs (Chernew et al, 1998; Westbrook and Braithwaite, 2010; Leite et al, 2020) in cases and in countries where the infrastructure functions well and technologies are supported by in-person care.

In an ideal world, combining data from different sources would allow patient care and overall health and social care to be applied in the delivery of care by the personnel. The costs of this ideal world, that is, online and data-driven care decision-making systems, are difficult to put against alternative cost structures. In fact, trying to distinguish the costs and the nature of care with or without technology is somewhat outdated (Keesara et al, 2020), as the examples of the pacemaker remote monitoring mentioned earlier, and care based on mobile sensors such as smartwatches or oxygen monitors, have been enabled with the development of specific surveillance technologies.

Even without the rapid and global COVID-19 crisis, technology as a remedy for the care crisis is not a straightforward solution, despite the investments. The new technology platforms are addressing citizens as consumers, and they have the potential to decrease some of the costs and increase some of the efficiency of care (for example Taylor et al, 2020). But not all technology platforms are used by citizen-consumers. The use of electronic health records (EHRs) in the US is still quite low, despite the investments (Wang and Huang, 2012). The personalised health records (PHRs) for citizen-consumers have not achieved the prediction of long-term usage in care either. Mobile health applications are designed to improve health-care delivery and communication between patients and hospitals, for example, but they are also used for informing patients of their appointments, among other features (Gagnon et al, 2016). While there is limited scientific evidence supporting the effectiveness of general mobile health monitoring, the number of health-related apps has increased globally from approximately 40,000 apps in 2012 to over 300,000 apps in 2019 (Mobile, 2020). Technology is thus also about a promise of delivery, not only about delivery.

Technology in social and health care can be used in a multitude of ways: the use ranges from mobile phone apps to time and separate the work tasks of nurses and home helpers, or sending home helpers to the next location, to monitoring and surveying workers, as in the Swedish home-care helpers' app use (Frennert, 2019). The division of home carers' work into smaller tasks that are measurable units means also that the recipients of care only get the kind of help that is articulated in those measurable terms, which is predetermined and predefined, and planned according to the requests and support item schemes. The care service work becomes 'taskified' (Kovalainen et al, 2020) with standardised and optimal time indications and time-paced service logics. It is indeed the case that the after-effects of Fordism are not dead, but have simply taken a new form in the transfer of timesheets used in industrial factories and assembly lines into mobile surveillance apps carried by workers. Timesheets are uploaded to care service workers' phones, pacing their work and service rhythm and care work in ways that are not visible to outsiders, but only to care recipients – and not even to the worker him/herself. The regulating power of the app is in its ability to compile data and use it in multiple ways.

Another aspect of technology in care are the gendered boundary conditions. By these, I refer here to the 'socioemotional' machines. Lucy Suchman's seminal analysis of the creation of human-like machines, where she analyses what becomes an imagined representation of humans through the eyes of roboticists (Suchman, 1987, 2003), gives an understanding of the use of gender stereotypes in standardising the human–robot interaction, thereby reproducing and reinforcing existing stereotypes (Weber, 2005).

Robots have become a well-established component of assisted living scenarios and smart-home scenarios for the near future. In most of these scenarios, the human–machine interface is a technology-based solution, a simplified idea targeted at easing everyday life and giving assistance to people in need of support. It is interesting that extensive research exists, such as about pet robots in day-care centres, nursing homes or residential care home settings (for example Preuss and Legal, 2017), but in these research papers, there is very little, if any, analysis of the aspects of the agency of elderly people, their willingness to adopt the technologies, or indeed, the sociality of machines and technologies. Sociality is interpreted to be an outcome of the interaction between individuals and not a feature of social life, and this then becomes transferred into robots (for example Sharkey, 2014).

Most studies on the use of robots in care lack reflective analysis of the methods used to gather and analyse research data, and instead new categorisations emerge. Weber (2005) has, for instance, distinguished between two kinds of interaction-relations in the human–robot interface that dominate, namely, the 'caregiver–infant relationship' and the 'owner–pet relationship'. This division obviously excludes health-care robotics such as exoskeletons, helping frail or paralysed persons to mobilise themselves, assistance in surgery, and monitoring and surveillance robotics, to mention but a few.

It is obvious that 'technology as remedy to care' discourses emerge not from the discourses of unpaid, informal, invisible, time-consuming and messy caring work, but from the discourses where care can be sliced into clear tasks that can be targeted for bids, and delivered, monitored and priced accordingly (Poutanen and Kovalainen, 2017). In a parallel manner, technologies of care receive attention as high-tech solutions such as assisting robots, and less when mobile phone care apps used by the home-care helpers are discussed.

It is estimated that roughly half the activities people are paid to do globally in current capitalism could be automated. Automation is not, however, straightforward but related to the complexity of transformation of production, reskilling and heterogeneity within occupations, for example (Vallas and Kovalainen, 2019; Kovalainen et al, 2020; Poutanen et al, 2020). It is important to ask, who are the users of technologies, and who are the beneficiaries of investments in technologies: is it the state, investors, citizen-consumers, or those who are being cared for? Some of the care work has already been automated and is among those activities to be in principle replaceable by technologies. Such technology is already in use in robot surgery and, for example, as assistive interpretation vehicles that do not merely help nurses or surgeons, but replace them (Coeckelbergh, 2012). In a similar manner, as medical technologies transform medical practices, also technologies within care, especially when ingrained into care work, monitoring and detailing care activities in work, also change the contemporary and prevailing care practices and processes, and undoubtedly also gradually transform the normative elements of what is understood as 'good care'.

Conclusion

Rather too easily, catch-all phrases such as neoliberalism and New Public Management are being brought in as the only or key explanations for the care crisis, whichever definition it is given, or to depict the uncertainties in care. Setting the historical context in place is a crucial aspect, as it calls for a deeper understanding of not only capitalism and its turns, but also the ways populism in politics turns into current actions manifested, among others, in the care crisis. This chapter has addressed some of the theoretical discussions, connected some discourses and critically reflected on the current care policies prevailing across the Nordic countries and beyond, where, for example, technology and the care crisis do not seem to easily meet. This chapter has offered insights into the point that care ethics, economics of care, technologies of care and politics are currently inseparable and tightly intertwined. These aspects are kept apart in academic discussions alike in much of the societal discussions.

As the discussions in this volume show, more nuanced gender analyses, for example, have to some extent been lacking, and unpaid care work is one of these fields. Unpaid care work makes a substantial contribution to most countries' economies, as well as to individual and societal well-being. How to address the care crisis discourses in ways that shed light on the complexity of struggles and persistence of inequalities that care work includes is highly needed.

There is also the need for real as opposed to virtual care, and for real as opposed to virtual social interaction. The development of robots for the care and companionship of older people increasingly opens up the possibility of meeting some of their needs by means of technology (Broekens et al, 2009; Borenstein and Pearson, 2010; Martin et al, 2015; Pillinger, 2019). As a 'remedy' to crisis, the various discussions seem to offer very different kinds of medicine as the question of the care crisis is not a one-dimensional question but a layered one that covers several aspects of care in society. Technology as a remedy and a promise of a remedy is justified mainly through the economic rationale that may carry constrained choices and may suppress several of the dimensions in the care crisis.

The tension between human work and technological aid in that particular work has been argued to diminish by building so-called 'moral machines' (Wallach and Allen, 2009). Automatisation is indeed rather naively being offered as a key remedy to care worker deficiency, but the practices prove otherwise, as studies among care workers' experiences with assistive technology show (for example Williams et al, 2014; Saborowski and Kollak, 2015). Technology has enabled the panopticon – omnipresence and measurement of all activities. More importantly, technology and digital care are seen as valuable economic assets that affect the process of care as 'value production'. The 'investments in technology of care' have replaced 'the investments in the care workers', and this has several gendered repercussions (Poutanen and Kovalainen, 2017).

The discourse analysis of globally influential policy documents, such as OECD documents, shows the ushering in of 'technology as remedy' and as a new paradigm and emerging frontier in which the development of health care and social care should be directed (Kovalainen, 2020). The promise of technology lies in its ability to enhance activities, from the selection of personalised care to the improvement of service delivery of that care. The potentialities of 'technology as remedy' are boundaryless, and in stark contrast to embodied care work and care provider costs with limited renewal and no scalable skills. Another part of the 'technology as promise and remedy' discourse is the enhancement of consumeristic citizenship through self-monitoring and self-management through their own health-care data. The disparities between socioeconomic groups in the use of technologies and digital illiteracy, or indeed the messiness of embodied care work are not cured by technology, however.

Finally, 'technology as remedy' relates seamlessly to the late-capitalist societies' state-level political decisions of innovation investments and production potentialities of technology that encompass all polities, care included. Most national innovation policies use technology as their springboard, and connect care with technology, but only at the level of innovation or industrial policy. And as much of the economies are built around high-tech industries, care services are only a logical extension to the development of new technologies and to the expansion of tech industries to new fields. For these reasons alone, the questions of the care crisis cut across the ethics of care, economics of care, politics of care and technologies of care, and presuppose alignments rather than detachments between these research fields.

Notes

[1] Private equity assumes cash flow and/or profitability. The valuation of private equity takes place solely through economic valuation, and assumes standardised and predictable activities, which are not often possible in care labour practices.

[2] Chapter 2 in this volume traces some of the key origins in feminist care literature by analysing self-reflexively the ways that the 'care crisis' has been attributed in articles by Phillips, Hochschild, Fraser and Williams.

References

Aglietta, M. and Breton, R. (2001) 'Financial systems, corporate control and capital accumulation', *Economy and Society*, 30(4): 433–466.

Ajunwa, I. (2017) Plenary talk at WORK2017 conference, University of Turku, Finland.

Anderson, B. and Shutes, I. (2014) 'Introduction' in B. Anderson and I. Shutes (eds) *Migration and Care Labour: Theory, Policy and Politics*, London: Palgrave Macmillan, pp 1–7.

Bedaf, S., Gelderblom, G.J. and de Witte, L. (2015) 'Overview and categorization of robots supporting independent living of elderly people: What activities do they support and how far have they developed', *Assistive Technology*, 27(2): 88–100.

Beedholm, K., Frederiksen, K. and Lomborg, K. (2016) 'What was (also) at stake when a robot bathtub was implemented in a Danish elder center: A constructivist secondary qualitative analysis', *Qualitative Health Research*, 26(10): 1424–1433.

Bodenheimer, T. (2005) 'High and rising health care costs. Part 2: Technologic innovation', *Annals of Internal Medicine*, 142(11): 932–937.

Borenstein, J. and Pearson, Y. (2010) 'Robot caregivers: Harbingers of expanded freedom for all?', *Ethics and Information Technology*, 12(3): 277–288.

Broekens, J., Heerink, M. and Rosendal, H. (2009) 'Assistive social robots in elder care: A review', *Gerontechnology*, 8(2): 94–103.

Çalışkan, K. and Callon, M. (2009) 'Economization, part 1: Shifting attention from the economy towards processes of economization', *Economy and Society*, 38(3): 369–398.

Chernew, M.E., Hirth, R.A., Sonnad, S.S., Ermann, R. and Mark, F.A. (1998) 'Managed care, medical technology, and health care cost growth: A review of the evidence', *Medical Care Research and Review*, 55(3): 259–288.

Coeckelbergh, M. (2012) '"How I learned to love the robot": Capabilities, information technologies, and elder care' in I. Oosterlaken and J. van den Hoven (eds) *The Capability Approach, Technology and Design*, Dordrecht: Springer, pp 77–86.

Coeckelbergh, M. (2015) 'Artificial agents, good care, and modernity', *Theoretical Medicine and Bioethics*, 36(4): 265–277.

Collins, S. (2015) *The Core of Care Ethics*, London and Basingstoke: Palgrave Macmillan.

Daly, M. and Lewis, J. (1998) 'Introduction' in J. Lewis (ed) *Gender, Social Care and Welfare State Restructuring in Europe*, Aldershot: Ashgate, pp 1–24.

Demiris, G. (2016) 'Consumer health informatics: Past, present, and future of a rapidly evolving domain', *Yearbook of Medical Informatics*, Suppl 1: S42–S47.

Dynan, K. and Sheiner, L. (2018) 'GDP as a measure of economic well-being', Hutchins Center on Fiscal and Monetary Policy at Brookings, Working Paper 43, Available from: www.brookings.edu/research/gdp-as-a-measure-of-economic-well-being. [accessed 15 June 2020].

Fraser, N. (2013) *Fortunes of Feminism: From State-Managed Capitalism to Neoliberal Crisis*, New York: Verso.

Fraser, N. (2014) 'Can society be commodities all the way down? Post-Polanyian reflections on capitalist crisis', *Economy and Society*, 43(4): 541–558.

Fraser, N. (2016) 'Capitalism's crisis of care', *Dissent*, 63(4): 30–37.

French, M. and Miller, F.A. (2012) 'Leveraging the "living laboratory": On the emergence of the entrepreneurial hospital', *Social Science & Medicine*, 75(4): 717–724.

Frennert, S. (2019) 'Lost in digitalization? Municipality employment of welfare technologies', *Disability and Rehabilitation: Assistive Technology*, 14(6): 635–642.

Gagnon, M.-P., Ngangue, P., Payne-Gagnon, J. and Desmartis, M. (2016) 'm-Health adoption by healthcare professionals: A systematic review', *Journal of American Medical Information Association*, 23(1): 212–220.

Gilligan, C. (1987) 'Moral orientation and moral development', reprinted in: Held, V. (ed) (1995) *Justice and Care: Essential Readings in Feminist Ethics*, Oxford: Westview Press, pp 31–46.

Hamington, M. (2015) 'Care ethics and engaging intersectional difference through the body', *Critical Philosophy of Race*, 3(1): 79–100.

Hampton, T. (2012) 'Recent advances in mobile technology benefit global health, research, and care', *JAMA*, 307(19): 2013–2014.

Held, V. (2006) *The Ethics of Care: Personal, Political and Global*, New York: Oxford University Press.

Horton, A. (2017) *Financialisation of Care: Investment and Organising in the UK and US*, PhD thesis, Queen Mary University of London, UK. Available from: http://qmro.qmul.ac.uk/xmlui/handle/123456789/31797 [accessed 15 July 2020].

Jorgenson, D.W. (2010) 'Designing a new architecture for the U.S. national accounts', *The Annals of the American Academy of Political and Social Science*, 631(1): 63–74.

Keesara, S., Jonas, A. and Schulman, K. (2020) 'Covid-19 and health care's digital revolution', *The New England Journal of Medicine*, 382(23): e82.

Kovalainen, A. (1999) 'The welfare state, gender system and public sector employment in Finland' in J. Christiansen, P. Koistinen and A. Kovalainen (eds) *Working Europe: Reshaping European Employment Systems*, Aldershot: Ashgate, pp 137–154.

Kovalainen, A. (2004) 'Rethinking the revival of social capital and trust in social theory' in B.L. Marshall and A. Witz (eds) *Engendering the Social: Feminist Encounters with Sociological Theory*, London: Open University Press, pp 151–171.

Kovalainen, A. and Österberg-Högstedt, J. (2011) 'Finland's changing public sector: Business, trust and gender in municipalities', *Nordiske Organisasjonsstudier*, 13(2): 57–73.

Kovalainen, A. and Sundin, E. (2012) 'Entrepreneurship in public organizations' in D. Hjorth (ed) *Handbook on Organizational Entrepreneurship*, London: Edward Elgar, pp 257–279.

Kovalainen, A., Vallas, S.P. and Poutanen, S. (2020) 'Theorizing work in the contemporary platform economy' in S. Poutanen, A. Kovalainen and P. Rouvinen (eds) *Digital Work and the Platform Economy: Understanding Tasks, Skills and Capabilities of the New Era*, New York: Routledge, pp 31–55.

Krippner, G.R. (2005) 'The financialization of the American economy', *Socio-Economic Review*, 3(2): 173–208.

Krippner, G.R. (2011) *Capitalizing on Crisis: The Political Origins of the Rise of Finance*, Cambridge, MA: Harvard University Press.

Le Grand, J. (1984) 'An introduction' in J. LeGrand and R. Robertson (eds) *Privatisation and the Welfare State*, London: Allen & Unwin, pp 1–12.

Le Grand, J. and Bartlett, W. (1993) 'Quasi-markets and social policy: The way forward?' in J. Le Grand and W. Bartlett (eds) *Quasi Markets and Social Policy*, Basingstoke and London: Macmillan, pp 202–220.

Leite, H., Hodgkinson, I.R. and Gruber, T. (2020) 'New development: "Healing at a distance"—telemedicine and COVID-19', *Public Money & Management*, 40(6): 483–485.

Levitsky, S.R. (2014) *Caring for Our Own: Why There Is No Political Demand for New American Social Welfare Rights*, Oxford: Oxford University Press.

Lusardi, A., Schneider, D. and Tufano, P. (2015) 'The economic crisis and medical care use: Comparative evidence from five high-income countries', *Social Science Quarterly*, 96(1): 202–213.

Martin, A., Myers, N. and Viseu, A. (2015) 'The politics of care in technoscience', *Social Studies of Science*, 45(5): 625–641.

Mayer, M.A., Rodríguez Blanco, O. and Torrejon, A. (2019) 'Use of health apps by nurses for professional purposes: Web-based survey study', *JMIR mHealth*, 7(11): e15195. doi:10.2196/15195

Menon, K. (2018) 'The state of care: Work, ethics and gender', *Contemporary Social Scientist*, 10(2): 23–30.

Mobile (2020) *Mobile Health Global Market Report 2013–2019: The Commercialization of the mHealth Applications*, Available from: www.globenewswire.com [accessed 12 January 2021].

Nieboer, M.E., van Hoof, J., van Hout, A.M., Aarts, S. and Wouters, E.J.M. (2014) 'Professional values, technology and future health care: The view of health care professionals in the Netherlands', *Technology in Society*, 39(C): 10–17.

OECD (Organisation for Economic Co-operation and Development) (2019a) *Health Care Quality Indicators*, OECD Statistics, Available from: www.oecd.org [accessed 10 March 2020].

OECD (2019b) *Health in the 21st Century: Putting Data to Work for Stronger Health Systems*, OECD Health Policy Studies, Paris: OECD Publishing.

Palm, E. (2013) 'Who cares? Moral obligations in formal and informal care provision in the light of ICT-based home care', *Health Care Analysis*, 21(2): 171–188.

Parreñas, R. (2001) *Servants of Globalization: Women, Migration and Domestic Work*, Stanford: Stanford University Press.

Peden, E.A. and Freeland, M.S. (1995) 'A historical analysis of medical spending growth, 1960–1963', *Health Affairs*, 14(2): 235–247.

Pillinger, A. (2019) 'Gender and feminist aspects in robotics', Working paper, Available from: http://www.geecco-project.eu/fileadmin/t/geecco/FemRob_Final_plus_Deckblatt.pdf [accessed 15 July 2020].

Pols, J. (2012) *Care at Distance: On the Closeness of Technology*, Amsterdam: Amsterdam University Press.

Pols, J. (2015) 'Towards an empirical ethics in care: Relations with technologies in health care', *Medicine, Health Care, and Philosophy*, 18(1): 81–90.

Pols, J. and Moser, I. (2009) 'Cold technologies versus warm care? On affective and social relations with and through care technologies', *ALTER, European Journal of Disability Research*, 3(2): 159–178.

Poutanen, S. and Kovalainen, A. (2017) *Gender and Innovation in the New Economy: Women, Identity and Creative Work*, New York: Palgrave Macmillan.

Poutanen, S., Kovalainen, A. and Rouvinen, P. (2020) 'Digital work in the platform economy' in S. Poutanen, A. Kovalainen and P. Rouvinen (eds) *Digital Work and the Platform Economy: Understanding Tasks, Skills and Capabilities of the New Era*, New York: Routledge, pp 3–9.

Preuss, D. and Legal, F. (2017) 'Living with the animals: Animal or robotic companions for the elderly in smart homes?', *Journal of Medical Ethics*, 43(6): 407–410.

Ratwani, R.M., Reider, J. and Singh, H. (2019) 'A decade of health information technology usability challenges and the path forward', *JAMA*, 321(8): 743–744.

Saborowski, M. and Kollak, I. (2015) ' "How do you care for technology?": Care professionals' experiences with assistive technology in care of the elderly', *Technological Forecasting and Social Change*, 93: 133–140.

Sampedro, V. (2011) 'Introduction: New trends and challenges in political communication', *International Journal of Press and Politics*, 16(4): 431–439.

Sandberg, B. and Elliott, E. (2019) 'Toward a care-centred approach for nonprofit management in a neoliberal era', *Administrative Theory & Praxis*, 41(3): 286–306.

Schiebinger, L. and Schraudner, M. (2011) 'Interdisciplinary approaches to achieving gendered innovations in science, medicine and engineering', *Interdisciplinary Science Reviews*, 36(2): 154–167.

Schillmeier, M. and Doménech, M. (2016) 'New technologies and emerging spaces of care: An introduction' in M. Schillmeier and M. Doménech (eds) *New Technologies and Emerging Spaces of Care*, London and New York: Routledge, pp 1–18.

Sevenhuijsen, S. (2004) 'Trace: A method for normative policy analysis from the ethic of care' in S. Sevenhuijsen and A. Schwab (eds) *The Heart of the Matter: The Contribution of the Ethics of Care to Social Policy in Some New EU Member States*, Ljubljana: Peace Institute, Institute for Contemporary Social and Political Studies, pp 13–46.

Sevenhuijsen, S., Bozalek, V., Gouws, A. and Minnaar-Mcdonald, M. (2003) 'South African social welfare policy: An analysis using ethics of care', *Critical Social Policy*, 23(3): 299–321.

Sharkey, A. (2014) 'Robots and human dignity: A consideration of the effects of robot care on the dignity of older people', *Ethics and Information Technology*, 16(1): 63–75.

Simonen, L. and Kovalainen, A. (1998) 'Paradoxes of social care restructuring: The Finnish case' in J. Lewis (ed) *Gender, Social Care and Welfare State Restructuring in Europe*, Aldershot: Ashgate, pp 229–255.

Suchman, L. (1987) *Plans and Situated Action: The Problem of Human–Machine Communication*, Cambridge: Cambridge University Press.

Suchman, L. (2003) *Human/Machine Reconsidered*, Lancaster: CSS, Lancaster University, Available from: www.comp.lancs.ac.uk/sociology/papers/Suchman-Human-Machine-Reconsidered.pdf [accessed 1 July 2020].

Taylor, C.B., Fitzsimmons-Craft, E.E. and Graham, A.K. (2020) 'Digital technology can revolutionize mental health services delivery: The COVID-19 crisis as a catalyst for change', *The International Journal of Eating Disorders*, 53(7): 1155–1157.

Timmerman, G., Baart, A. and Vosman, F. (2019) 'In search of good care: The methodology of phenomenological, theory-oriented "N=N case studies" in empirically grounded ethics of care', *Medicine, Health Care and Philosophy*, 22(4): 573–582.

Tronto, J. (1995) 'Care as a basis for radical political judgments', *Hypatia*, 10(2): 141–149.

Tronto, J. (2010) 'Creating caring institutions: Politics, plurality and purpose', *Ethics and Social Welfare*, 4(2): 158–171.

Vallas, S.P. and Kovalainen, A. (2019) 'Introduction: Taking stock of the digital revolution' in S.P. Vallas and A. Kovalainen (eds) *Work and Labor in the Digital Age*, New York: Emerald, pp 1–12.

Vogel, S.K. (2018) *Marketcraft: How Governments Make Markets Work*, Oxford: Oxford University Press.

Walker, M.U. (2007) *Moral Understandings: A Feminist Study in Ethics* (2nd edn), Oxford: Oxford University Press.

Wallach, W. and Allen, C. (2009) *Moral Machines: Teaching Robots Right from Wrong*, Oxford: Oxford University Press.

Wang, C.J. and Huang, A.T. (2012) 'Integrating technology into health care: What will it take?' *JAMA*, 307(6): 569–570.

Weber, J. (2005) 'Helpless machines and true loving care givers: A feminist critique of recent trends in human–robot interaction', *Journal of Information, Communication and Ethics in Society*, 3(4): 209–218.

Wenzlaff, F. (2019) 'Economization of society: Functional differentiation and economic stagnation', *Journal of Economic Issues*, 53(1): 57–80.

Westbrook, J. and Braithwaite, J. (2010) 'Will information and communication technology disrupt the health system and deliver on its promise?', *Medical Journal of Australia*, 193(7): 399–400.

WHO (World Health Organization) (2014) *Economic Crisis, Health Systems and Health in Europe: Impact and Implications for Policy*, Available from: www.euro.who.int/__data/assets/pdf_file/0008/257579/Economic-crisis-health-systems-Europe-impact-implications-policy.pdf [accessed 10 August 2020].

Williams, A., Goodwin, M. and Cloke, P. (2014) 'Neoliberalism, Big Society, and progressive localism', *Environment and Planning A*, 46(12): 2798–2815.

Williams, F. (2011) 'Towards a transnational analysis of the political economy of care' in R. Mahon and F. Robinson (eds) *Feminist Ethics and Social Policy: Towards a New Global Political Economy of Care*, Vancouver and Toronto: University of British Columbia, pp 127–144.

Wilson, M. (2002) 'Making nursing visible? Gender, technology and the care plan as script', *Information Technology & People*, 15(2): 139–158.

Wouters, O.J. and McKee, M. (2017) 'Private financing of health care in times of economic crisis: A review of the evidence', *Global Policy*, 8(2): 23–29.

Yeates, N. (2009) *Globalizing Care Economies and Migrant Workers: Explorations in Global Care Chains*, Basingstoke: Palgrave.

Yeatman, A. (2018) 'Gender, social policy and the idea of the welfare state' in S. Shaver (ed) *Handbook on Gender and Social Policy*, London: Edward Elgar, pp 21–36.

5

Deteriorating working conditions in elder care: an invisible crisis of care?

Anneli Stranz

Introduction

The Nordic welfare states are often described as 'potentially women-friendly' due to the availability of publicly provided services that support women to combine paid work and caring responsibilities. While such services reduce the extent of informal care tasks and increase the possibilities of labour market participation for large groups of women, paid elder care workers have often been neglected in this narrative of women-friendliness (Theobald, 2003; Dahl, 2004). Therefore, care workers face the risk of being invisible in the feminist dialogue concerning a 'care crisis'. Recurring reports on the problematic work situation in Swedish elder care (for example Work Environment Authority, 2015, 2020), calls for analyses of care workers' position in society and what is needed in terms of redistribution of material needs and institutional recognition to achieve *gender justice* (Fraser, 2007).

Long-term care for older adults is generally characterised by austerity, cost-cutting and new market-inspired models of governance in the public sector (Rostgaard et al, 2012; Deusdad et al, 2016). These wide-ranging trends and changes in the public sector influence women generally because they are the primary users of many of the state benefits, and women tend to fill the gaps of state withdrawal by providing additional informal care (Anttonen, 1990). Women are also affected as paid workers, since the public sector is highly staffed by women. Within the Nordic labour market and the rest of the Anglo-Saxon world, frontline care staff are part of a low-status, low-paid and low-skilled group (Waerness, 1984; England, 2005; Weir, 2005; Razavi and Staab, 2010; Newman, 2017). In paid care work, women are the 'default caregivers' (Penz and Sauer, 2017).

Nine out of ten elder care workers in Sweden are women and moreover gender is also essential when it comes to who uses elder care services: twice as many women as men aged 65+ receive elder care services in Sweden (NBHW, 2019). Thus, women form the majority of both care workers and care recipients. Elder care is hence an exceedingly gendered issue and a feminist approach is desirable to understand how different dimensions of care interlink in a time of immense changes that will transform the elder care sector in the coming decades. High levels of retirement, difficulties in recruiting and retaining care workers and a higher proportion of old persons in the population put pressure on the 'caring welfare state', characterised by an ambition of universalism and a passion for equality (Szebehely and Meagher, 2018). A key question in the near future is who will care for the old and what are the costs for paid care workers?

Elder care is an important social infrastructure in the Nordic welfare states and therefore highly important for almost all citizens in different phases of life. These different stakeholders – care recipient, care worker and informal carer – are hugely influenced in their everyday life by changing legislation, care policies and reorganisations. To state an example, care workers need adequate working conditions to have a good work life and be able to give care recipients the care they need and are entitled to. Further, informal carers need to trust the quality of public care to be able to share the care burden with professionals (the welfare state) and/or be able to have full-time work. An older person's possibility to affect their daily life is reliant on these factors. In each of these three groups, women are in the majority and as a result are living the consequences of changing social policies. Tonkens et al (2013: 407) note that 'welfare state reform is a source of high drama in people's lives, entailing significant emotional costs and efforts to cope with its impact'.

Several studies on care work have shown that the organisation of elder care services have a direct impact on everyday care work performed and what quality of care that is possible to give (Meagher et al, 2016; Stranz and Sörensdotter, 2016). However, changes in policies and reorganisations in elder care in Sweden have not been adapted to the frontline care workers' experiences and skills. The everyday realities of practical care work and the important fact that the work is intellectual, emotional and relational have seldom been highlighted or considered in the restoration of the care sector (James, 1992; Stranz and Szebehely, 2018). These circumstances depict care workers as highly neglected; several care researchers have pointed out invisibility and lack of voice as a common feature of the paid care worker's everyday work life (Grugulis and Vincent, 2009; Dahl, 2010; Banerjee et al, 2015).

When identifying and theorising the concept of *care crisis* in the Nordic context, an important factor is to investigate how women in different social positions are influenced by structural changes concerning social care. This chapter will focus on an often-excluded group, elder care workers, which constitute a very large group in the female-dominated labour market. The aim of the chapter is to study and analyse Swedish elder care workers' experience of their working conditions by using survey data. The work situation is framed within a model built on a two-dimensional approach to gender justice (Fraser, 2007).

Theoretical approach

Researchers with a feminist approach have underscored that revaluing care work is an essential factor of any struggle for a just society (for example, Tronto, 1993, 2017; Stone, 2000; Kittay, 2005; Dahl, 2010; Fraser, 2016). However, it is not an easy assignment to point out what is needed to revalue paid care work in welfare societies. It will probably involve a combination of reforms on different levels, from micro- to macro levels as they are intertwined.

The theoretical perspective adopted in the chapter is Fraser's (2000, 2007) *two-dimensional justice model*, which builds on an overarching principle of *parity in participation*, a condition where the social arrangements permit all members of society to interrelate as peers. In order to achieve the condition of parity in participation, the society needs to take action with a focus on both material and economic redistribution and actions that weaken status inequality (Fraser, 2000, 2007).

Fraser's two-dimensional model of justice critiques the traditional division between recognition and redistribution, which are viewed as two forms of justice that cannot be brought together (Fraser, 2000; Fraser and Honneth, 2003). In the dual model of justice, the aim is to treat recognition as a question of social status. This means that it is the individual group members' status as full participants in social interaction that requires recognition. Status inequality in this model is understood as embedded in institutionalised patterns of cultural value, which establish some actors as inferior (Fraser, 2000; Fraser and Honneth, 2003).

The aim of treating recognition as social status is to overcome this subordination by establishing the devalued group as fully represented in the community. Fraser (1997) here responds to mainstream multiculturalism and the affirmative remedies for such injustices, that proposes to redress disrespect by revaluing unfairly devalued group identities. In contrast, transformative remedies are associated with deconstruction and thus enable the possibility to change the status of devalued groups by redistributing material resources that guarantee all participants independence and voice (Fraser, 2000).

Thus, misrecognition and unfair distribution are rooted in different forms of injustice; accordingly, the means for addressing them differ. Unfair distribution involves some form of economic restructuring, such as redistribution of income, reorganisation of the division of labour or transformation of other basic economic organisation. Status inequality, on the other hand, requires deinstitutionalising patterns of cultural value that impede equality of participation (Fraser, 1996, 2000).

Moreover, Fraser (2000) assumes that the category of gender holds both political and economic dimensions, as it is a basic structuring principle of society (Table 5.1). Gender constitutes the dividing line between paid *productive*

Table 5.1: A two-dimensional conception of gender

Gender	
Redistribution	Recognition
Political economy:	Status subordination:
Productive-reproductive	Devalues femininity
Division of labour	
Gender-specific forms of maldistribution	Gender-specific forms of misrecognition

Source: Fraser (2000, 2007)

work and unpaid *reproductive work*, and the division of wage labour. This relation results in political and economic structures that create gender-specific forms of mistreatment and marginalisation. Gender also encodes the cultural interpretations and value patterns that are central to a society, which manifests itself in what is referred as androcentrism (devaluation of the feminine). As a result, both perspectives, as illustrated in Table 5.1, focus on an important aspect of women's subordination. Fraser states (2007: 26) that 'It is an open question whether the two dimensions are of equal weight. But rectifying gender injustice, in any case, requires changing both the economic structure and the status order of contemporary society. Neither, alone, will suffice'.

A central starting point in this chapter is the assumption that paid care work is part of a gender-segregated labour market and, consequently, is devalued because of its connection to femininity. The aim is to use the dimensions of recognition and redistribution concurrently, and in doing so enable comprehension of the interaction between the dimensions. Fraser's examples (1996, 2007) of how to apprehend the concept of *gender justice* often bear reference to the structural level (for example, policies and legislation). The intention of this chapter is to also make use of the model on a micro level with examples from everyday care work. The overall research question is: How can we understand the care crisis with the care workers' experiences of working conditions as a point of departure?

Trends in Swedish elder care: ageing-in-place, deinstitutionalisation and decreased service coverage

The Nordic countries share several features and general trends regarding the organisation of the elder care system. In an international comparison, the Nordic countries are generous when it comes to public spending on social services, including elder care. However, a decline in coverage has taken place in all countries and a focus on ageing-in-place instead of institutional care is a prominent feature, as in many other Western societies (Deusdad et al, 2016).

In Sweden, between 1980 and 2015, the service coverage dropped and the proportion of the population aged 80+ receiving home-based or residential care reduced from 62 per cent to 37 per cent. In the 1980s and 1990s, the decrease started in home care but more recently it is the coverage in residential care that has declined considerably. Between 2000 and 2015, one-quarter of residential care beds disappeared and the proportion of the population aged 80+ in residential care decreased from 20 per cent to 13 per cent (NBHW, 2019). In the same period, the number of home-care users increased but the rise has probably not compensated for deinstitutionalisation as hardly any home-care user receives the same extent of care as in residential care (Ulmanen and Szebehely, 2015).

Another significant change concerns how elder care is organised and provided. Since the beginning of the 1990s, market-inspired principles have transformed both the organisation and provision of publicly financed welfare services, particularly in elder care (Erlandsson et al, 2013). These principles were implemented in all Nordic countries but to varying degrees, with Sweden and Finland being more affected than Denmark and Norway. These changes, inspired by New Public Management (NPM), are characterised by a purchaser–provider split, competition, standardisation, auditing and accountability (Anttonen and Meagher, 2013).

Further, partly as a consequence of marketisation and quality control, staff face increased demands to document the care they give to the care recipient so that data are available on what actually was done (Stranz and Szebehely, 2018). This trend is reinforced by the focus on person-centred care, which is stressed in legislation and national policy (Government Report, 2017). For each client, the assessment by the case manager is written down in a care plan that contain the resident's needs, habits and preferences, and care workers are supposed to regularly update these plans. Another form of documentation concerns checklists and non-conformance reports. Both care workers and their managers thus spend increasing amounts of time on documentation of various kinds, and these work tasks have escalated over time (Stranz and Szebehely, 2018).

One further highly important and ongoing change is the altering needs of the care recipients. Policies accentuating 'ageing-in-place' and a trend of deinstitutionalisation lead to an increasing number of older people with extensive needs living at home, and consequently an older and frailer population living in residential care homes (Schön et al, 2015). A result of the decline in coverage is an increase in family care.

The process of marketisation, with a focus on branding, and the more complex needs among care recipients have once again put the question of education on the agenda. Although the requirements for trained personnel, meaning nurse assistants, are emphasised in national policies and local guidelines. Due to a deficit of care workers, municipalities in Sweden have to hire unskilled staff (often by the hour) to provide elder care. Currently, 45 per cent of employees are working by the hour and 20 per cent of permanent employees lack relevant education (Government Report, 2019). Therefore, there is a discrepancy between the political requirements for educated staff and the fact that employers hire persons with a lack of relevant training. Further, labour shortages have led to a turn to migrant recruitment and an increasing proportion of the care workforce are migrants (28 per cent) (NBHW, 2019).

According to the Health and Social Care Inspectorate (IVO, 2018), the lack of education is one of the causes of the maltreatment affecting care recipients. Moreover, several reports have focused on the escalating problems involving the insufficient language skills, which complicates communication between different stakeholders in everyday care work (Government Report, 2019).

Working conditions in elder care: a Nordic outlook

The problematic and arduous working conditions in female-dominated welfare occupations cannot be understood as a new occurrence. Both health-related issues and problems of recruiting and retaining care workers have been investigated in Swedish government commissions and reports over the years. Additionally, current reports from the Swedish Work Environment Authority provide a picture of increasing work-related problems, and notifications of occupational disease due to social and organisational causes have increased over the last decade. These notifications are often related to psychosocial working conditions, in particular to relationships in the workplace such as difficult contacts with clients, threats and violence, and lack of support from managers and colleagues (Work Environment Authority, 2015, 2020).

Even though the Nordic social service model is characterised as recognising paid care work through state obligation and professionalisation (Dahl, 2010), there is a continuous deterioration of care workers' job quality, characterised by factors such as high bodily and mental demands, time strain and it being harder to give the care needed (Trydegård, 2012).

The Nordcare study, a postal survey questionnaire administered to care workers in the Nordic countries in 2005 and 2015, displays a general trend of deteriorating working conditions in elder care in all the Nordic countries (Rostgaard and Matthiessen, 2016; Szebehely et al, 2017; Kröger et al, 2018; Strandell, 2020). Norway is the only country where the working situation has not deteriorated as much as in the other Nordic countries between the years 2005 and 2015. However, there are differences between the countries as well, and Sweden stands out as having a more problematic work situation when it come to some central aspects of the work environment. Firstly, in both Sweden and the rest of the Nordic countries, the proportion of care workers who want to leave their work increased over the 2005–2015 period. However, both in 2005 and 2015, a higher share of the respondents (50 per cent in the year 2015) in Sweden wanted to quit their job. The combined percentage for the other three countries is 39 per cent. Moreover, the increase in the proportion of respondents who almost always feel physically and mentally tired after a day's work increased in all Nordic countries between 2005 and 2015. In Sweden, however, the increase is more evident and can be defined as a critical case when unfolding a care crisis (Szebehely et al, 2017). Additionally, among Swedish care workers as well as Finnish and Danish care workers, there is a major reduction in decision latitude (especially in home care) and a substantial increase in having too much to do at work (especially in residential care homes) (Szebehely et al, 2017).

Data and analysis

The analysis is based on the Nordcare study, a survey sent to care workers in the Nordic countries in 2005 and 2015. In 2005, a mail questionnaire was distributed to 5,000 unionised care workers in home and residential settings (overall response rate: 72 per cent). In 2015, a similar questionnaire was sent to 8,000 elder care workers in the Nordic countries (response rate: 55 per cent). Since approximately eight of ten Swedish care workers are unionised, the sample is representative of the care workforce, although those with the most precarious employment conditions are underrepresented (Szebehely et al, 2017). The survey instrument included both open-ended and closed questions covering aspects such as employment qualifications, organisation of care, working conditions, content of the working day and workers' experiences of their paid work.

This chapter presents the results from a qualitative analysis of open-ended questions from the Swedish part of the Nordcare study from 2015. Both care aides and assistant nurses, working in home care and residential care, are included in the analyses. The qualitative analyses were conducted using the guidelines of a directed content analysis, with theory or prior research used to further investigate the area of knowledge (Hsieh and Shannon, 2005). This meant identifying and condensing meaning units, coding and categorising, and this process started by inputting and analysing all the responses in Statistical Package for the Social Sciences (SPSS). Secondly, the respondents' answers to the open-ended question were imported to NVivo Pro 11.4, which was used to conduct the qualitative analyses. The answers to the question, *if you think you will quit your job now or in the future, please state why*, were merged into a single text document in the software. The resulting data are not connected to individuals or different workplaces. The coding process was related to the quantitative analyses of the Nordcare survey data already conducted (see Szebehely et al, 2017; Stranz and Szebehely, 2018; Strandell, 2020) and also inspired by earlier research on care work as a welfare service and practice with a focus on working conditions.

Results

The presentation of the results that follows is categorised in six themes that illustrates gender-specific working conditions related to both maldistribution and misrecognition: unsatisfying employment conditions; work–life imbalance; lack of resources; physically and mentally demanding; relational poverty; and endangered well-being.

With reference to the *two-dimensional model of justice* the results (categories) are understood as containing both an economic and institutional dimension. To paraphrase Fraser, it is important to have in mind that it is important to look at both dimensions simultaneously. Thus, every category of working conditions presented is understood to comprise both a dimension of redistribution and recognition and that both aspects are highly interwoven and non-excluding (Fraser, 2007).

Unsatisfying employment conditions

Low income is a matter of high concern for the respondents in the Nordcare study. The most common statement in this category is that the wages are far too low in relation to the responsibilities they have at work. Another aspect mentioned is that the low wages reflect the low status connected to care work. The following quotes highlight the intrinsic tension between status and wages:

> That the salary and status of this profession is despicable; the society shows whom and what matters and it is not us working with people.

> Poor working hours and poor pay, tough with all the stress and no one is thanking for the work we do.

Furthermore, the respondents find their employment conditions unsatisfactory. Some of the care workers would need to work more hours to get by economically, and others want a permanent position and the security that comes with this.

> Can't get full-time employment; instead I work extra hours when someone is on sick leave or on vacation.

It is an obvious problem that care workers have a low salary and cannot get full-time employment; this is a salient feature in women-dominated work sectors. Additionally, part-time work is more common in elder care than in other sectors of the Swedish labour market, which is also the case in other women–dominated domains (Stranz and Szebehely, 2018). More than half of the elder care workers in Sweden work part-time, often involuntarily as they are not offered full-time work or in response to a demanding work situation (Meagher et al, 2016). The option to have employment conditions that live up to the androcentric norm of productive work is not available for the responding care workers (Fraser, 1994).

Work–life imbalance

Among the respondents who are parents, some express dissatisfaction with the working hours, especially in the evenings and at weekends. These quotes illustrate that the schedules existing in elder care are not easily compatible with life outside work:

> Working hours fit poorly with home life.

> The schedule, I want to find a workplace where the working hours fit parents of young children, to keep the family together.

Employers seems to plan and reorganise the schedules with a focus on labour intensity rather than considering the care workers' need to organise family life or offering recovery from strenuous work. Another development regarding work time is that an increasing number of care workers have to work every other weekend.

> It is difficult to get together with my family when I work every other weekend.

Further, split shifts (when work time is divided into two shifts with a longer unpaid break in between) have become a widespread method of organising working hours in Sweden. Results from the Nordcare study (Szebehely et al, 2017) show that one in ten care workers have split shifts every week; this pattern of employment is more common in residential care homes than in home care. In the other Nordic countries, only a small percentage of care workers work split shifts at all. According to the respondents this way of organising work time influences both quality of life and family life in a negative manner.

Lack of resources

The care workers in the survey often refer to lack of resources when describing the physically heavy work in elder care. The most prominent aspect described is that there are too few staff, which contributes to an almost permanent lack of time.

> Tiring job, tired of the staffing level being too low, too many work tasks to do in a day, a lot of responsibility.

The staffing level in elder care is an important issue when it comes to the quality of care. In comparison with other care regimes, Sweden is generous in this aspect (Harrington et al, 2012). However, the phenomenon of working with inadequate staffing levels is well documented in empirical studies on care work in Sweden (Stranz, 2013), and it seems that staff experience this phenomenon continuously. Even if the staffing ratio is adequate on the schedule, it is usual practice that vacations, sick leave and so on are not filled in (Szebehely et al, 2017).

> Because there is a high level of staff shortages, sick leaves every day, too high work rates, we are going to keep up with more and more tasks without getting more time or staff.

A relevant staffing level is a prerequisite for achieving continuity in relations, flexibility regarding how to plan the day and a possibility of adapting to continually shifting and individual needs and wishes of care recipients. The everyday organisation of care work is thus strained in a way that contradicts some of the core values of working with older persons with complex needs: enough time, sufficient decision latitude and continuity in relations. Understaffing highlights the institutional devaluation of care as intellectual and emotional work. However, the care workers must do the same amount of work as usual, even when they are short-staffed. This is an obvious lack of recognition as the definition of what working as a care aid or nurse assistant encompasses seems to be boundless, changing from time to time. The role of the skilled care worker is negotiated and deconstructed based on different structural and organisational needs with little discretion for the care workers to influence their situation. The illimitable increase of work tasks and a permanent lack of staff is not noted in relation to wage remuneration.

Physically and mentally demanding

The experience of a too-heavy workload is a salient feature in everyday care work and embraces both mental and physical aspects of working conditions. Examples from the open-ended question reveal responses noting not just a high physical or mental workload, but that these aspects of everyday work are intimately intertwined. As demonstrated, the statements testify to a high work pace that gives rise to stress among respondents.

Moreover, lack of time can also result in a situation where heavy tasks such as lifting are executed in incorrect positions and at a faster tempo. In the literature, care work is repeatedly described as physically demanding (for example Trydegård, 2012), which is also revealed in the results. Some care workers describe why they have thoughts of leaving work, such as the following:

> Due to heavy lifting, incorrect work positions, one-sided work.

> It's hard, the insufficient staffing takes my energy, wears on my back and body; the job is exhausting.

Experiences of mental strain is often expressed in terms of feeling constant stress, illustrated in the following quotes:

> Because I cannot handle the stress as it is now.

> Stress, a bad manager, I am almost a robot.

Some care workers also emphasise their worries of forgetting important work tasks due to time constraints.

> Physically and mentally demanding, afraid to forget things with users, feel I cannot cope with an increasing work pace.

Another experience described with regard to the amount of work is the continuous increase in the number of work tasks (such as documentation), which can result in a sense of working conditions gradually getting worse. Unwanted work tasks (such as cleaning and washing) are also described as stealing time from more important chores. This can be understood in relation to the characteristic of the organisation of care work in Sweden: the care workers collectively engage in most work tasks independent of their occupational position or educational background (Szebehely, 2017). The following quotes illustrate this conflict between too many different work tasks and wishes to socialise with the care recipient.

> The stress, too much documentation, would like to spend more time of my working hours with the elderly, not all the documentation that just increases.

> The workload is constantly increasing ... less time for the residents. Cleaning and laundry is more important than the residents are. There is no time to sit down with residents who need a moment of conversation.

The described feelings of stress and too much to do seem to partly be a conflict between different categories of work tasks. Several studies have shown that care workers perceive the interpersonal aspects of work as the core of caregiving. Tasks that 'take time from the resident' are generally described as tasks that should not be included in their work (compare Banerjee et al, 2015). The concept of 'illegitimate tasks' has recently been introduced in the literature as a current workplace stressor, and is defined as work tasks that violate the worker's role identity (Björk et al, 2013). Consequently, it is described as a signal from the employer that encodes a lack of appreciation and undermines the worker's self-esteem.

Relational poverty

Care research has pointed out that good relations, which include the possibility to fully attend to the care recipient's requests, make the work meaningful and are also a motivation for care workers to stay at their workplace (Dybbroe, 2012; Stranz, 2013). In their answers, staff describe continuous feelings of not being able to respond to the care recipients' bodily, emotional, relational and social needs:

> The customers are not getting the help they need. When you feel that you have not done a good job, you feel bad.

> I do not feel that I can do a good job and I see that the residents are suffering a lot from this.

> It is because I can't give the care that my care recipients or users deserve and because we are so controlled by the minute; stress, stress.

The depicted conditions make it difficult for the staff to feel satisfied with the help they give: in other words, the users do not always get the care they need. The lack of time makes the staff stressed and they have to struggle to give good care. Feelings of inadequacy can be further explained using the concept of moral distress. The care workers try hard to give the users good-enough care, but their efforts are not valued: resources are scarce and the tasks they need and want to perform are invisible. Feelings of inadequacy and distress in relation to the care recipient has been shown to be a risk for care workers' health (Trydegård, 2012).

Endangered well-being

The care workers' statements about the job being both emotionally and physically heavy often relate to the experience of their own well-being.

Health-related issues are a prominent reason for not being able to stay in the elder care sector. The physical workload is a problem both in relation to an already worn-out body and to the fact that they also express worries about the future and whether their bodies can handle the increasing demands.

> Too heavy work, have pain in the body; it is exhausting both physically and mentally. I have worked in elder care for 25 years and now I am 63 years old and will retire earlier. Sore legs and back; after many years in social care my body is worn out.

> My body is ageing; you get older and can't take it because of the workload and not enough staff.

> Too heavy work, have body pain; the work is demanding both physically and mentally.

> Almost everyone quit at my workplace eventually because of pain and injury from work.

In these examples, the care workers describe their health in a way that irradiates the significance of a healthy body to cope with everyday work in elder care: the staff's bodies are obviously a central working tool. The result of a too-heavy workload can be a worn-out body and this can force staff to quit; it might not be a choice. A worn-out body might also affect the quality of life in a negative way after retirement. Experiencing physical and mental tiredness after a work shift contributes to a slow process of wear and tear, which, without satisfying recovery, can lead to serious health problems (Aronsson et al, 2010; Sonnentag et al, 2017). The bodies of the care workers are central in their daily work but time pressure, lack of staff and heavy workload have escalated in the last decades and most certainly reinforced the institutional misrecognition of care and care work (Stranz and Szebehely, 2018).

Conclusion

The aim of the chapter was to investigate how care workers in Swedish elder care experience their working conditions by analysing an open-ended question, from the Nordcare survey, concerning possible reasons to quit their job now or in the future. The overall research question was whether we can study the *care crisis* with the care workers' everyday work experiences as a point of departure. Additionally, two dimensions of justice – recognition and redistribution – were used concurrently to illuminate the interaction between the two dimensions, referring to the following themes: insufficient employment conditions; work–life imbalance; lack of resources; physically and mentally demanding; relational poverty; endangered well-being.

To sum up, the care workers find it hard to support themselves economically and the organisations' inflexibility underpins an imbalance between paid work and life outside work. The respondents have to work in understaffed workplaces because of scarce resources, and the effect is stress and being unable to provide good care in line with the service users' needs as well as political ambitions. Moreover, the work is both physically and mentally arduous and the respondents report having excessive problems with bodily and mental fatigue. The definition of care work as intellectual, emotional and relational clashes with the conditions of work evolving from the analyses in the present study. The care workers' experience of stress and mental plus physical exhaustion are not compatible with daily encounters with persons in need of care and support. Consequently, the staff are put in a position where they are forced to prioritise which work tasks are the most immediately important, due to a far too arduous working situation.

From a two-dimensional perspective of justice, the work situation for Swedish care workers undermines the status of care work through unfair distribution of economic and material goods and institutional devaluation. The aspects of work presented all relate to the care workers' thoughts of leaving their job, which can be interpreted as a highly important issue for achieving attractive working conditions at a time of a 'recruitment crisis'. Further, the themes evolving from the everyday work can be assumed as encompassing both gender-specific redistribution and misrecognition, referring to the structural assumption that paid care work is part of a gender-segregated labour market and, consequently, devalued because of its connection to reproduction and femininity.

The chapter has provided some examples of how the two-dimensional model can be used to analyse working conditions as experienced by the care workers. Not many people would question the claim that work in elder care is low paid and it is a common assumption that higher pay would increase the status of the profession. But to assume that the salary itself would create these changes is not likely from this theoretical point of view. This is because it is basically also about *why* the wages increase. To deconstruct the picture of care work, the institutional valuation needs to be considered: is there additionally an intention to make work tasks and skills visible 'as work'?

Further, lack of resources – especially low staffing levels – is a permanent condition in the care-providing organisation, and thus in the everyday work. These concerns are accentuated through institutional devaluation, the time needed to do the work is undistinguishable and staff need to adapt to the staffing level, which can fluctuate from day to day. The work is done anyway but probably the price is high, especially in the long run when the body cannot take it anymore. As a result, workers have restricted influence on how to claim for more resources.

Consequently, the present crisis of care workers' situation, including lack of resources, reproduces unfair economic and material distribution and misrecognition at both the micro and macro levels and strengthens injustice based on gender stereotypes. The dimension of gender, as women are in the majority both as care workers and care recipients, needs to be highlighted in social policies that concern elder care, since social policy influences people's everyday lives and communicates what is possible or not, and what is high status or not. The consequences for older persons in need of care, mainly women, is rarely discussed as a gender issue, and for that reason need to be emphasised in research and policy.

If the required political reforms do not take place, care workers will remain in a vulnerable position, and neglected as full participants in the institutional settings of society and in the distribution of economic resources. It is hard to imagine how the welfare states will deal with ongoing and upcoming challenges such as ageing societies and problems in recruiting and retaining staff. This is a current and accelerating 'crisis of care' with gender inequality as the core characteristic.

However, the COVID-19 pandemic has changed the map, at least temporarily. Massive infection outbreaks and deaths in Swedish elder care, especially residential care homes, have put the elder care sector and current weaknesses under the spotlight (Szebehely, 2020). As a response to the critical situation in Swedish elder care at the start of the pandemic, the Swedish prime minister Stefan Löfven proclaimed in an interview (Sveriges Radio, 2020): 'We all [political parties] agree that we need to equip the elder care sector with safer employment conditions, more colleagues and with additional education.'

The situation calls for a reorganisation of the infrastructure of elder care focusing on how to allocate resources and responsibilities. Perchance the COVID-19 crisis, which has affected a large proportion of citizens, will help to highlight the low institutional status and silenced voices of care workers and citizens in need of elder care services.

Struggles for better working conditions were introduced by assistant nurses before the pandemic with warnings about the situation in elder care. In August 2019, an organisation called 'undersköterskeupproret' (the struggle of care workers) started demonstrations all over the country to campaign for improved working conditions. The assistant nurses handed over 14,500 signatures to social minister Lena Hallengren. The care workers declared that they want to be able to combine work with social and family life. They do not want to be worn out and risk long-term sick leave because of the pressured workload and feelings of inadequacy in relation to the users. They also need more colleagues, with the right skills (Kommunal, 2019). In

October 2019, five months before the outbreak of COVID-19 in Swedish residential care homes began, the same group, 'undersköterskeupproret', warned the government that economic cutbacks will lead to chaos in elder care (ETC, 2019): 'We do not require any increased wages, only more colleagues, in order to avoid the stress that eventually cause the body to break.'

This substantial organisation of care workers included in 'undersköterskeupproret' and the recognition they received from the politicians did not lead to a redistribution of resources. However, 'undersköterskeupproret' and their message were partly recognised by politicians for example by a structured meeting with the social minister and also by the media. But, the efforts did not lead to any clear result. However, the political intention was noticeably not to redistribute resources to elder care and the action made it impossible to disrupt the fundamental institutional structure that endlessly produces injustice. The kind of recognition obtained was 'affirmative' with no clear ambition to transform the two dimensions of justice concurrently (Fraser, 1997).

Sustainable elder care characterised by *gender justice*, with the power to divert the *crisis of care*, has to offer improved employment and working conditions that facilitate the care workers' possibility to work without becoming mentally and bodily exhausted and risking their well-being. Additionally, the work situation in elder care needs to be continually related to users, a majority of whom are women, receiving elder care. The highly problematic work situation, at a time of recruitment crisis and with the users having increasingly complex needs, is of course a significant challenge for a welfare state with the ambition to provide high-quality care to all citizens. The political as well as organisational ambitions of giving older persons influence and participation in their daily life can almost certainly not be achieved under these conditions of work.

Improved working conditions, beginning in the everyday micro processes, with a focus on both equal distribution of economic and material needs, as well as institutional recognition, can support an upgrading of care work and make the problematic aspects of the working conditions in elder care visible, and possible to mend. At that point, it will be possible to move the transformations forward, away from deepening the care crisis; otherwise, the position of care workers, and consequently care users, will become enduringly degraded in society.

References

Anttonen, A. (1990) 'The feminization of the Scandinavian welfare state' in L. Simonen (ed) *Finnish Debates on Women's Studies*, Tampere: University of Tampere, Research Institute for Social Science, pp 3–49.

Anttonen, A. and Meagher, G. (2013) 'Mapping marketisation: Concepts and goals' in G. Meagher and M. Szebehely (eds) *Marketisation in Nordic Elder care*, Stockholm: Stockholm University, pp 13–21.

Aronsson, G., Astvik, W. and Gustafsson, K. (2010) 'Arbetsvillkor, återhämtning och hälsa – en studie av förskola, hemtjänst och socialtjänst', *Arbete och hälsa*, 44(7): 1–34.

Banerjee, A., Armstrong, P., Daly, T., Armstrong, H. and Braedley, S. (2015) '"Careworkers don't have a voice": Epistemological violence in residential care for older people', *Journal of Aging Studies*, 33: 28–36.

Björk, L., Bejerot, E., Jacobshagen, N. and Härenstam, A. (2013) 'I shouldn't have to do this: Illegitimate tasks as a stressor in relation to organizational control and resource deficits', *Work & Stress*, 27(3): 262–277.

Dahl, H.M. (2004) 'A view from the inside: Recognition and redistribution in the Nordic welfare state from a gender perspective', *Acta Sociologica*, 47(4): 325–337.

Dahl, H.M. (2010) 'An old map of state feminism and an insufficient recognition of care', *NORA*, 18(3): 152–166.

Deusdad, B.A., Pace, C. and Anttonen, A. (2016) 'Facing the challenges in the development of long-term care for older people in Europe in the context of an economic crisis', *Journal of Social Service Research*, 42(2): 144–150.

Dybbroe, B. (2012) 'Perspectives: A daily conflict of creating and losing meaning in elder care' in H. Hvid and A. Kamp (eds) *Elder care in Transition: Management, Meaning and Identity at Work: A Scandinavian Perspective*, Copenhagen: Copenhagen Business School Press, pp 133–159.

England, P. (2005) 'Emerging theories of care work', *Annual Review of Sociology*, 31: 381–399.

Erlandsson, S., Storm, P., Stranz, A., Szebehely, M. and Trydegård, G.-B. (2013) 'Marketising trends in Swedish elder care: Competition, choice and calls for stricter regulation' in G. Meagher and M. Szebehely (eds) *Marketisation in Nordic Elder care*, Stockholm: Stockholm University, pp 23–75.

ETC (2019) 'Undersköterskeupproret varnar – nedskärningarna ger kaos', Available from: www.etc.se/ekonomi/underskoterskeupproret-varnar-nedskarningarna-ger-kaos [accessed 15 September 2020].

Fraser, N. (1994) 'After the family wage: Gender equity and the welfare state', *Political Theory*, 22(4), 591–618.

Fraser, N. (1996) *Social Justice in the Age of Identity Politics: Redistribution, Recognition and Participation*. The Tanner Lectures on Human Values. Delivered at Stanford University, 30 April to 2 May 1996.

Fraser, N. (1997) *Justice Interrupts: Critical Reflections on the 'Post Socialist' Condition*, New York: Routledge.

Fraser, N. (2000) 'Rethinking recognition', *New Left Review*, 3(May/ June): 107–120.

Fraser, N. (2007) 'Feminist politics in the age of recognition: A two-dimensional approach to gender justice', *Studies in Social Justice*, 1: 23–35.

Fraser, N. (2016) 'Contradictions of capital and care', *New Left Review*, 100(July/August): 99–117.

Fraser, N. and Honneth, A. (2003) *Redistribution or Recognition? A Political–Philosophical Exchange*, London: Verso.

Government Report (2017) *Läs mig! Nationell kvalitetsplan för vård och omsorg för äldre personer*, Stockholm: Ministry of Health and Social Affairs, Available from: https://www.regeringen.se/rattsliga-dokument/statens-offentliga-utredningar/2017/03/sou-201721/ [accessed 15 September 2020].

Government Report (2019) *Stärkt kompetens i vård och omsorg*, Available from: www.regeringen.se/rattsliga-dokument/statens-offentliga-utredningar/2019/04/sou-201920/ [accessed 15 May 2020].

Grugulis, I. and Vincent, S. (2009) 'Whose skill is it anyway? "Soft" skills and polarization', *Work Employment and Society*, 29(4): 597–615.

Harrington, C., Choiniere, J., Goldmann, M., Jacobsen, F.F., Lloyd, L., McGregor, M., Stamatopoulos, V. and Szebehely, M. (2012) 'Nursing home staffing standards and staffing levels in six countries', *Journal of Nursing Scholarship*, 44(1): 88–98.

Hsieh, H.F. and Shannon, S.E. (2005) 'Three approaches to qualitative content analysis', *Qualitative Health Research*, 15(9): 1277–1288.

IVO (2018) *Vad har IVO sett 2018? Iakttagelser och slutsatser om vårdens och omsorgens brister för verksamhetsåret 2018*, Available from: www.ivo.se/publicerat-material/nyheter/nyheter-2019/vad-har-ivo-sett-2018---risker-och-brister-i-vard-och-omsorg/ [accessed 15 September 2020].

James, N. (1992) 'Care = organisation + physical labour + emotional labour', *Sociology of Health & Illness*, 14(4): 488–509.

Kittay, E.F. (2005) 'Dependency, difference and the global ethic of long-term care', *The Journal of Political Philosophy*, 13(4): 443–469.

Kommunal (2019) 'Undersköterskeupproret kräver bättre arbetsvillkor och fler utbildade kollegor', Available from: https://blogg.kommunal.se/utredare/2019/08/22/underskoterskeupproret-kraver-battre-arbetsvillkor-och-fler-utbildade-kollegor/ [accessed 10 August 2020].

Kröger, T., Van Aerschot, L. and Puthenparambil, J.M. (2018) 'Hoivatyö muutoksessa: suomalainen vanhustyö pohjoismaisessa vertailussa', *YFI julkaisuja*, 6.

Meagher, G., Szebehely, M. and Mears, J. (2016) 'How institutions matter for job characteristics, quality and experiences: A comparison of home care work for older people in Australia and Sweden', *Work, Employment & Society*, 30(5): 731–749.

NBHW (National Board of Health and Welfare) (2019) *Vård och omsorg om äldre. Lägesrapport 2019*, Available from: www.socialstyrelsen.se/globalassets/sharepoint-dokument/artikelkatalog/ovrigt/2019-3-18.pdf [accessed 3 October 2020].

Newman, J. (2017) 'Re-gendering governance in times of austerity: Dilemmas of feminist research, theory and politics' in C. Hudson, M. Rönnblom and K. Teghtsoonian (eds) *Gender, Governance and Feminist Analysis: Missing in Action?* New York: Routledge, pp 35–52.

Penz, O. and Sauer, B. (2017) 'Affective governmentality: A feminist perspective' in C. Hudson, M. Rönnblom and K. Teghtsoonian (eds) *Gender, Governance and Feminist Analysis: Missing in Action?* New York: Routledge, pp 39–58.

Razavi, S. and Staab, S. (2010) 'Underpaid and overworked: A cross-national perspective on care workers', *International Labour Review*, 149(4): 407–421.

Rostgaard, T. and Matthiessen, M.U. (2016) *Arbejdsvilkår i ældreplejen: Mere dokumentation og mindre tid til social omsorg*, København: KORA.

Rostgaard, T., Timonen, V. and Glendinning, C. (2012) 'Guest editorial: Reforming home care in ageing societies', *Health & Social Care in the Community*, 20(3): 225–227.

Schön, P., Lagergren, M. and Kåreholt, I. (2015) 'Rapid decrease in length of stay in institutional care for older people in Sweden between 2006 and 2012: Results from a population-based study', *Health and Social Care in the Community*, 24(5): 631–638.

Sonnentag, S., Venz, L. and Casper, A. (2017) 'Advances in recovery research: What have we learned? What should be done next?', *Journal of Occupational Health Psychology*, 22(3): 365–380.

Stone, D. (2000) 'Why we need a care movement', *The Nation*, 13 March: 13–15.

Strandell, R. (2020) 'Care workers under pressure: A comparison of the work situation in Swedish home care 2005 and 2015', *Health & Social Care in the Community*, 28(1): 137–147.

Stranz, A. (2013) *Omsorgsarbetets vardag och villkor i Sverige och Danmark: ett feministiskt kritiskt perspektiv*, PhD thesis, Stockholm: Stockholm University.

Stranz, A. and Sörensdotter, R. (2016) 'Interpretations of person-centered dementia care: Same rhetoric, different practices? A comparative study of nursing homes in England and Sweden', *Journal of Aging Studies*, 38: 70–80.

Stranz, A. and Szebehely, M. (2018) 'Organizational trends impacting on everyday realities: The case of Swedish elder care' in K. Christensen and D. Pilling (eds) *The Routledge Handbook of Social Care Work Around the World*, London: Routledge, pp 45–58.

Sveriges Radio (2020) Interview with Swedish Prime Minister Stefan Löfven, 20 June.

Szebehely, M. (2017) 'Residential care for older people: Are there lessons to be learned from Sweden?' *Journal of Canadian Studies*, 50(2): 499–507.

Szebehely, M. (2020) 'COVID-19 reveals serious problems in Swedish long-term care', Available from: https://ltccovid.org/2020/05/08/covid-19-reveals-serious-problems-in-swedish-long-term-care/ [accessed 17 August 2020].

Szebehely, M. and Meagher, G. (2018) 'Nordic elder care: Weak universalism becoming weaker?' *Journal of European Social Policy*, 28(3): 294–308.

Szebehely, M., Stranz, A. and Strandell, R. (2017) *Vem ska arbeta i framtidens äldreomsorg?* Working Paper 2017:1, Stockholm: Stockholm University, Department of Social Work.

Theobald, H. (2003) 'Care for the elderly: Welfare system, professionalization and the question of inequality', *International Journal of Sociology and Social Policy*, 23(4–5): 159–185.

Tonkens, E., Grootegoed, E. and Duyvendak, J.W. (2013) 'Introduction: Welfare state reform, recognition and emotional labour', *Social Policy and Society*, 12(3): 407–413.

Tronto, J. (1993) *Moral Boundaries: A Political Argument for an Ethic of Care*, New York: Routledge.

Tronto, J. (2017) 'There is an alternative: Homines curans and the limits of neoliberalism', *International Journal of Care and Caring*, 1(1): 27–43.

Trydegård, G-B. (2012) 'Care work in changing welfare states: Nordic care workers' experiences', *European Journal of Ageing*, 9(2): 119–129.

Ulmanen, P. and Szebehely, M. (2015) 'From the state to the family or to the market? Consequences of reduced residential elder care in Sweden', *International Journal of Social Welfare*, 24(1): 81–92.

Waerness, K. (1984) 'Caring as women's work in the welfare state' in H. Holter (ed) *Patriarchy in a Welfare Society*, Oslo: Universitetsforlaget, pp 67–87.

Weir, A. (2005) 'The global universal caregiver: Imagining women's liberation in the new millennium', *Constellations*, 12(3): 308–330.

Work Environment Authority (2015) *Sociala och organisatoriska orsaker*, Korta arbetsskadefakta Nr 6, Stockholm: Arbetsmiljöverket.

Work Environment Authority (2020) *Projektrapport, Äldreomsorgen 2017–2019. Riskfylld arbetsmiljö – utmaningar för framtidens äldreomsorg*, Stockholm: Arbetsmiljöverket.

6

Managerialism as a failing response to the care crisis

Hanna-Kaisa Hoppania, Antero Olakivi, Minna Zechner and Lena Näre

Introduction

For several decades now, elder care services have been characterised by recurring crises in Finland. In 2006, a political scandal erupted when allegations became public of insufficient staff ratios in Koukkuniemi, the largest unit of institutional care for older adults in the Nordic countries at the time (Yle, 2006). In 2019, a scandal broke when the National Supervisory Authority for Welfare and Health (Valvira) ordered the closure of several care homes owned by private care companies due to severe neglect in the quality of care, and announced that they were investigating several complaints regarding deficiencies in elder care (Valvira, 2019). Valvira's lawyer described the situation in the first care home as an 'acute crisis', which is why it was closed down immediately (Tiessalo, 2019). The situation was described as a 'care crisis' by the media, expert commentators and opposition politicians as well as the Regional State Administrative Agencies (AVI, 2020).

Care crisis is understood here as referring to a situation in elder care that has reached a critical phase in relation to the quality of care, also involving public concerns over the quality and conditions of care work. While a crisis is commonly understood as a temporary disruption, for many people in the world, such as older adults in poor health, a crisis can become a lasting, endemic condition. Nevertheless, when a crisis has been identified by central actors in the field, action needs to be taken.

In Finland, a common line of action is routinely suggested as a solution to the crisis of elder care: improvements in the management of care. When developments and outcomes in elder care turn into a media frenzy and draw public attention to deficiencies and problems of all kinds from individual neglect and abuse to systematic understaffing, poor working conditions and widespread inadequate and inhumane treatment, at some point, the quality of management is identified as a key factor causing the strife, and hence better management is proposed as a solution to the crisis (for example Räsänen, 2011; Hoppania, 2015; Hoppania et al, 2017). However, very little public debate has emerged about what (good–quality) care management actually entails. How, precisely, can management solve the acute problems in the quality of care and care work? Why do the crises of care persist, after years of intensive efforts to resolve them by improvements in management? This chapter approaches these questions by bringing the recent research on management trends in elder care into dialogue with theories of the logic and rationality of care.

The chapter begins by discussing management trends in the care sector since the 1980s to 1990s. While many of these trends are global, the discussion focuses on the Nordic countries and Finland in particular, with an empirical focus on home care and institutional elder care. Firstly, a brief discussion is provided of the historical and argumentative context in which management has emerged as a key target of political intervention. Managerialism, as a belief and value system that stems from the world of business and production rather than reproduction, has emerged as the driving ideology in the reform of elderly care in Finland and beyond.

Secondly, the chapter explores two prevailing trends of management as they have emerged in elder care in Finland. Drawing on Hanne Marlene Dahl (2009), the discussion distinguishes between the predominantly rationalistic *logic of details* as a systemic logic that shapes the structures of care provision, and the more normative *logic of self-governance* as an affectively appealing discourse that offers emotionally engaging subjectivities and (often false) optimism to floor-level care management in various organisations. These trends have been the object of care research to an extent, notably in the work of Dahl (2009, 2012; also, Hoppania et al, 2017; Olakivi, 2018; Hirvonen et al, 2020), and in a number of empirical case studies discussed in this chapter. The contribution to the existing literature is to examine these two sides of managerialism explicitly in light of the *logic of care* (Mol, 2008).

The logic of care focuses on the needs of the individual and on care relationships. Since care needs are situational and temporal, they are seldom similar even for individuals of the same age and with the same illness. Instead, care needs vary even for the same person at different times. The production of care differs from, say, the production of cars and toothbrushes. This creates evident complications in the context of increasingly marketised care, including in Finland where private companies have dramatically increased their share of care provision during the past three decades (Karsio and Anttonen, 2013; Kröger, 2019). The marketisation of care, together with the increasing influence of business consultants in public service provision (Hirvonen et al, 2020), has also shaped publicly owned care organisations by introducing management styles that are imitating industry and business. These managerial styles have influenced the work of women in particular, who comprise a great majority of care workers all over the world. Men, in turn, are over-represented in the higher echelons of managerial hierarchies, also in the care field (Adams, 2010; Hussein et al, 2016).

After discussing the different trends of management in light of the logic of care, the chapter returns to the socio-political context of the care crisis and the pitfalls of managerialism that have been exposed. Neither of these management styles sufficiently respect the logic of care, and at worst they contribute to the production of new crises. Moreover, it appears that the political focus on management obscures the root cause of the care crisis: the under-resourcing and undervaluing of gendered and embodied professional care work.

Quality and efficiency through management?

According to Kröger (2019), a demographic panic has been driving Finnish care policies, and governments have put a great deal of effort into avoiding their constitutional responsibility to serve the care needs of older adults. The avoidance of this responsibility has predominantly been implicit, with little open political discussion about the responsibilities of care (Hoppania, 2015), before the supervising bodies closed care homes and media coverage became widespread in 2019. Incremental changes, such as more stringent needs testing and rises in client fees have led to complicated service systems and difficulties in accessing services. The politics of avoidance have created a situation in which family members need to shoulder heavier responsibilities than before, and the numbers of reports and complaints about inadequate care have increased dramatically, especially since 2019 (AVI, 2020). Another crisis is located within care work, characterised by staff shortages and employees' psychophysical overload (Kröger et al, 2018).

Public debate and policy routinely offer better management as a solution to the crises (for example, STM, 2017). The alluring idea is that good management limits the need for economic investments in public care provision (Hoppania, 2015). This argument was strong even in the 1980s and 1990s during the first wave of New Public Management (NPM) that made the management of service provision a key target of political intervention (Henriksson and Wrede, 2008; Hoppania et al, 2016). In practice, NPM entailed management styles and tools from the private sector and businesses being implemented in the public sector, including in the provision of elder care (Trydegård, 2012). NPM has been an international project, where ideas have travelled across countries and sectors. As a result, care work management in Finland and beyond has borrowed management styles, for example, from Japanese car factories (Lean Management), the US navy (Total Quality Management) and big business (Balanced Scorecards) with diverse results (Trydegård, 2012; Hirvonen et al, 2020).

NPM has been infused with high hopes, but also criticised (Diefenbach, 2009). According to critics, the constant focus on the development of management has diverted attention away from other targets of development, such as inadequate staff ratios and the fact that people with intensive care needs are increasingly forced to live at home. Indeed, the question about sufficient resources has typically been sidelined in elder care policy reforms, even if it has somewhat paradoxically been the driving force behind those reforms (Hoppania, 2015). This might be changing now in Finland, at least to some extent, as in 2020 the parliament committed to raising staff ratios in care homes – albeit only gradually and excluding home care services. Nevertheless, research suggests that currently the Finnish care system is in 'a situation where, as a result of both individual and structural issues, [older] people in need of care do not receive sufficient assistance from informal or formal sources, and thus have care needs that remain uncovered' (Kröger et al, 2019: 3). In comparison to the level of funding for elder care services in other Nordic countries, Finland is over one billion euros short annually (Seppälä, 2019). When public officials responsible for elder care in the municipalities were asked about the sufficiency of home care, nearly one in two (46 per cent) replied that there are not enough home care services (THL, 2018). Clearly the enduring political focus on the development of care management has not solved these problems in Finland.

The diversifying toolbox for managing care work

Managerialism refers to a broad ideology of industrialised societies according to which problems in almost any area of society can be effectively resolved via managerial interventions (Räsänen and Trux, 2012: 45; Klikauer, 2015). Managerialism can be seen as an ideology whereby the world gets better when it is put into the hands of specialised managers (Räsänen and Trux, 2012: 42). The aim is to control people and issues and ignore what cannot be controlled. From a managerialist perspective, moreover, management is a specific job, a profession requiring specific training and skills (Grey, 1999). Managerial skills are specific, but they allegedly apply to any field of work. As Thomas Klikauer (2015: 1107) writes: 'Managerialism's perilous central doctrine is that differences between a university and a car company are less important than their similarities and that the performance of all organisations can be optimised by the application of generic management skills and knowledge.' Resisting managerial interventions, and interventions by business consultants promoting the latest trends of managerialism, may be particularly difficult for female-dominated service occupations, including elder care work, compared to male-dominated fields, such as medicine (Hirvonen et al, 2020).

In Finland, care work managers (including leaders, supervisors and middle managers) are still expected to have specific training for care work and not only for management. However, management has become a new and independent field of expertise and a target for development and improvement in care work. Hence, while managers aim to manage care work, the work of managers is a target of management as well. New management styles, models, ideals and structures are developed continuously – and care work managers are expected to develop themselves accordingly.

The turn to managerialism is a relatively recent one in care work in Finland. During the heyday of Nordic welfare state politics (1970–1990), Finnish care politics placed a relatively strong emphasis on professional – instead of managerial – ideals and ethics of care provision (Henriksson et al, 2006). According to the professional ideals, care workers and their supervisors should have a relatively highly specialised and formal education in care work and their activities should primarily follow professional ethics of care (Paasivaara, 2002). These ideals have by no means lost their power in Finland: legislatively, care workers and their supervisors are still required to have formal education in care (Act on Qualification Requirements for Social Welfare Professionals, 272/2005). In comparison to other Nordic countries, Finnish care workers have the highest educational levels (Kröger et al, 2009). Since the early 1990s, however, political debates in Finland have become increasingly critical of professionalism in care (Henriksson and Wrede, 2008). Critical arguments have depicted professional care systems as old-fashioned, self-serving, economically inefficient, inflexible and not transparent enough (Henriksson and Wrede, 2008). To solve these problems, critics routinely call for better management. The increasing marketisation of care, and the respective diversification of public and private care providers, has only increased the calls for transparency and managerial control (for example Sitra, 2018).

Political and public calls for transparency, flexibility, efficiency and quality can be difficult to object to (Dahl, 2012). Yet care workers and academic commentators have criticised managerial transformations, especially transformations that imitate a specific style of management: the industrial and Taylorist model of standardised work processes, hierarchical planning, and formalised surveillance and control systems of care workers, originally developed for factory work management (Dahl, 2009; Diefenbach, 2009).

Contemporary working life tends to idealise innovations, flexibility and self-governing employees – in contrast to Taylorist standardisation. While few nowadays openly advocate Taylorism in elder care management, a number of Taylorist management tools have been implemented in care work since the 1990s. These include the obligation of care workers to constantly document and report on their work – an obligation that has been resisted by care workers since the 1990s (Paasivaara, 2002). Another Taylorist tool is the creation of quasi-markets within public care production, including the idea according to which care provision can be disintegrated into standardised, measurable and statistically comparable products and routines that care workers – especially in home care – perform by following pre-planned timetables and to-do lists (Heikkilä et al, 2014). These practices draw on an industrial management ideology that Dahl (2009) calls the logic of details.

The logic of details also implies new divisions of labour in care work. Professionals in leadership roles are increasingly expected to act as specialised managers in charge of the detailed control of their staff members' performance – rather than as experienced seniors who offer guidance to their junior colleagues (Bolton, 2005; King, 2012). This division of labour mitigates the importance of professional care work skills, education and specialisation both among managers and frontline workers. Instead of skilled professionals, the logic of details requires a flexible, compliant and controllable workforce willing to work according to the instructions and timetables planned by higher-level managers (Henriksson et al, 2006). To increase flexibility, a shorter educational path to the most routinised jobs in elder care work has been established under the title of care assistant in Finland (Sinervo et al, 2013). Moreover, this division of labour enables high turnover rates in care: if care workers mainly follow timetables and plans imposed on them by others, and require less work expertise and experience, they become increasingly replaceable. Often employers find such replaceable care workers among migrants and racialised minorities, especially in the metropolitan region of Helsinki (Näre, 2013; Olakivi, 2019). In Helsinki, 24 per cent of care assistants were foreign-born in 2016 (Statistics Finland, 2019). The proportion of foreign-born care assistants has more than tripled from 2004 (7 per cent), while the proportion of foreign-born care managers has remained close to zero (Statistics Finland, 2019).

The Taylorist logic of details is not the only trend of Western managerialism in contemporary societies (Miller and Rose, 2008). Taylorist management has also become a common target of critique in care work (Gilbert, 2005; King, 2012). The ideology of managerialism has had to constantly renew itself and seek new legitimacy. Compared to the Taylorist principles of standardisation, hierarchy and external control, prevailing managerial trends tend to highlight almost opposite values, such as innovation, flexibility and employees' internal control (Boltanski and Chiapello, 2005). In recent decades, such managerial ideals and arguments have, to a degree, travelled from business and industrial management to public service provision (O'Reilly and Reed, 2010). In line with Dahl (2009), this chapter argues that these managerial trends draw on the logic of self-governance.

The logic of self-governance expects care workers to be responsible, autonomous, proactive, self-steering and reflexive agents who constantly develop themselves, solve problems in their organisational environments and get things done – regardless of burdensome and precarious working conditions (Moffatt et al, 2014; Olakivi, 2017). The logic of self-governance expects care work managers, in turn, to activate and empower these qualities in their subordinates. Instead of hierarchical controllers of the Taylorist model, care work managers are expected to act as inspiring leaders (O'Reilly and Reed, 2010), facilitators (du Gay et al, 1996), motivational coaches (Oldenhof et al, 2016) or 'enterprising co-ordinators of care' (Bolton, 2005: 8), who influence their subordinates via subtle human resource management techniques (such as performance appraisal interviews and the articulation of 'organisational values').

Theoretically, the logic of self-governance sits well with the traditional, professional ideals of Finnish welfare state politics. While there is a clear conflict between professional ideals and the Taylorist logic of details, the logic of self-governance, to a degree, aligns with the professional ideals of internal devotion, responsibility and constant development (O'Reilly and Reed, 2010; Olakivi and Niska, 2017; see also Chapter 8 in this volume). The logic of self-governance can, however, also impose novel expectations on care workers and their managers: instead of highlighting formal and specialised education for care work, professional traditions and collective responsibility, the logic of self-governance highlights generic creativity, learning by doing, and the constant comparison of individual workers with respect to their personal performance and productivity (Moffatt et al, 2014; Olakivi, 2017).

Both lines of care work management, the logic of details and the logic of self-governance, are associated with the *neoliberal* politics of public welfare provision (Dahl, 2009). Whereas the logic of details highlights hierarchies and external standardisation, the logic of self-governance highlights another aspect of the neoliberal project (Miller and Rose, 2008; Baines et al, 2012): it conceives personal responsibility and constant self-development as solutions to structural problems. In Finnish private and public sectors, publicly funded development projects according to the logic of self-governance have gained economic and ideological support since the 1990s (Arnkil, 2004; Hirvonen et al, 2020).

However, the growing appeal of the logic of self-governance has not led most care organisations to abandon the logic of details. Rather, care organisations have adopted some of the ideals of self-governance alongside the prevailing logic of details and the ideals of external control, disintegration and fragmentation. Many care organisations continue to implement information technologies and relatively faceless systems of reporting, recording and monitoring as management tools for streamlining processes by comparing separate units' performance statistics (Ahosola and Lumme-Sandt, 2019). Respectively, the same organisation can have a number of middle managers and lower-level supervisors (ward managers, head nurses, home care supervisors) who have little control over the top-level management systems and technologies (Björk et al, 2013). The main task of these supervisors and middle managers is to coach, inspire, motivate and activate their subordinates' commitment, attitudes and values, and abilities to govern themselves and manage their jobs regardless of the Taylorist system (Antonsson, 2013). In this task, the discourse of self-governance can offer middle managers affectively appealing resources, tools and subjectivities – but, as we move on to argue, it can also create novel conflicts between care workers and their supervisors.

The logic of care and the limits of detailed control

Care is a particular kind of practice that follows the logic and rationality of its own (Waerness, 1984; Mol, 2008). The logic of care means that – unlike on the factory floor, or in clearly defined service products such as haircuts – the needs that require a response can change rapidly and unexpectedly. Care involves a human relationship in which the response of the one receiving care plays a part (Fisher and Tronto, 1990; Anttonen and Zechner, 2011). Care, at least good care, is an ongoing process including the care-giver and care-receiver rather than a defined service product (Mol, 2008; Zechner, 2008).

The starting point in care work is always the need for care, not choice or want. In professional care work, the worker has to recognise and understand the kind of care that is required in a particular situation, and also to respect the autonomy of the person in need of care. Care is always about bodily, corporeal relationships. Individual caring situations are indirectly affected by a complex network and history of care relations. The personal (care) histories of the care-giver and the care-receiver affect the situation and both parties' experiences of it (Valokivi and Zechner, 2009; Hoppania et al, 2016).

Paying attention to the bodily dimension of care illustrates the psychic and material limits of detailed care management (Twigg et al, 2011). One can never be certain how a body will respond to care. Similarly, since care is relational work, the cognitive and emotional responses of both the person in need of care and the care worker vary (King, 2012). Care is always unpredictable to an extent, and therefore care work that follows the logic of care requires sensitivity and the ability to respond to changing situations. Hierarchical attempts to standardise and control care in line with the logic of details cause problems precisely due to this logic's incompatibility with the logic of care (Hoppania and Vaittinen, 2015).

A key source of conflict between the logic of details and the logic of care derives from time use. Implementing economic rationalisation in care work that ontologically resists standardisation is bound to make conceptions of time collide. The Taylorist logic of details gives care workers few opportunities to adjust their work rhythms to the changing situations (Astvik and Melin, 2012). For example, defining and standardising the amount of time that particular tasks for the recipients of care – such as eating, bathing, giving medication – should take, a common practice especially in home care in Finland, ignores the logic of care and the unpredictable nature of care situations. This can decrease both the quality of care and care workers' well-being and satisfaction, as care workers' abilities to follow the ethics of care dramatically decrease (Hirvonen and Husso, 2012). When managerially standardised time frames of work conflict with the actual time frames of care, a further danger is that the workers' needs – that is, their needs to satisfy their employers but also to take care of their own well-being in precarious working conditions – start to compete with the needs of the recipients of care (Sipiläinen et al, 2011). In Finnish home care, 39 per cent of employees state that in order to get their work done, they need to contravene the principles or rules of the workplace (Vehko et al, 2017).

According to a common argument, the logic of details pursues both economic efficiency and quality of care. In this view, the quality of care improves if organisations have more control over the services they offer, by monitoring the performance and time use of care workers and the conditions of the recipients of care, and by collecting detailed information that higher-level managers and experts can quantify and statistically compare. These practices of rational-technical (Trevithick, 2014) quality control effectively ignore the everyday experience and professional knowledge of care workers, and also of middle managers and lower-level supervisors, in favour of higher-level management, numerical data and controlled methods.

Numerical data can, of course, be useful when different units and care organisations are compared. Ideally, numerical data can uncover real problems and highlight successes in the quality of care. It is, however, far from self-evident that numerical data can measure all aspects of the quality of care and the actual, situationally changing needs of the care recipients (Kurunmaki et al, 2016). In Finland, the long-lasting interest in numerical quality control has not prevented recurring crises. At worst, the logic of details can create separate realities: one in the everyday life of care, practical needs and encounters; another in the systems of higher management in which the recipients of care as well as care workers are reduced to numbers that are managed from a distance (Hoppania et al, 2016).

Finally, continuous reporting and monitoring of care absorbs time from actual care work. According to a recent study from Finland (Kröger et al, 2018), the proportion of elder care workers that considered that documentation consumed too much of their working time grew from 38 per cent in 2005 to 70 per cent in 2015. Paradoxically, the tool that was meant to control the quality of care can duly become an impediment to good care (Banerjee, 2013).

Organisations and service systems can tackle these problems if they start to understand care as a human relationship and professional work that follows the ethics and logic of care. Consequently, the possibilities of management appear in a different light: what is central to management and policy-making is to create conditions that enable work practices in line with the logic of care where individual and situational needs for care direct the organisation of care work. To enable this, care workers must have professional ethics and skills, including formal education, and practical abilities to form lasting relationships with their care recipients. Lasting relationships are a precondition for care workers to be able to recognise situational changes in the needs of the recipients of care. Growing turnover rates in elder care work hamper this precondition. Finally, care workers must have practical resources – that is, time – to respond to the care recipients' situational, changing and unpredictable needs.

The logic of care and the limits of self-governance

In the 2020s, the inadequacy of Taylorist management is relatively well acknowledged in Finland among care workers, academics and also among middle managers and lower-level supervisors in old age care. The ways in which middle managers and care work supervisors understand and talk about good care often follow the logic of care instead of the logic of details (Stenman et al, 2015). These understandings highlight the importance of respecting older persons' individual needs and the need to invest time in the interaction between care workers and the recipients of care (Surakka et al, 2014: 225–226). How middle managers can progress from appreciating the logic of care discursively to supporting it in practice is, however, another question.

In care work organisations, middle managers inhabit a difficult position. If the larger structural systems of care follow the Taylorist logic of details, and if middle managers lack the power to transform these structures, their options are limited. Yet managerial discourses expect middle managers to have an impact on care, and these discourses are normatively compelling (Olakivi, 2018). Middle managers can find the subjectivities enabled by the logic of self-governance affectively appealing and empowering (Olakivi and Niska, 2017). Instead of transforming the external systems of care work organisation – that may seem impossible – managers can conceive of themselves as inspiring leaders and motivational coaches (O'Reilly and Reed, 2010; Oldenhof et al, 2016; Hirvonen et al, 2020). They can activate their subordinates in becoming more responsible and independent actors able to proactively and dynamically respond to the care recipients' unpredictable needs, regardless of the Taylorist structures. In an article by Olakivi and Niska (2017: 27), a head nurse in a Finnish public sector care home described her work, as a 'coach', as follows:

> What I find most difficult is maybe giving negative feedback, or if we have to give warnings. That's not nice. I prefer being like a coach. So

that I support and try to find a way so that the people will find the right way to act and find their own strengths, and that way support the functions as well.

The logic of self-governance seems to offer new optimism for care work managers. According to the optimist ideal, care work managers do not have to force their subordinates to act against the ethics of care. Instead, they can coach their subordinates to serve these ethics, but in alignment with more distant and less visible socio-political and economic objectives (Hirvonen et al, 2020) – that is, the political objective to avoid economic investments in the material conditions of care work. This management style aims to translate the objectives of employers and policy-makers – better economic efficiency – into projects more easily acceptable to care workers – better quality of care and constant self-development (Moffatt et al, 2014). Simultaneously, the care worker is detached from their social relationships and brought under the managerial gaze as an individual target of intervention, with individual values, emotions and self-management abilities as targets of development. In the article by Olakivi and Niska (2017: 28), a home care supervisor discussed elder care work, its burdens, and her own reactions to these burdens, as follows:

> It's a bit like you either like it [care work] or you don't. So in my opinion, when people always talk about the rush, the rush is a bit self-imposed [by care workers], so that sometimes you even have to stop people and go, like, 'Hey, would you just sit down and see that it's not really that bad after all'.

Solving problems in care work via the logic of self-governance is not easy. Firstly, care organisations' support for employees' self-governance often seems superficial. If the structures of care continue to be organised according to the Taylorist logic of details, and if care workers are not granted the actual autonomy to decide how they organise their daily work, or the education and experience to enable such decisions, expecting care workers to govern themselves may appear to be a tall order – or simply another form of exploitation (Olakivi, 2018). Care workers are mainly given the autonomy to decide how they navigate through the plans, timetables and obligations imposed on them by others (Boyd, 2002). Supporting self-governance turns into supporting care workers' sense of responsibility, not their autonomy. If these techniques of coaching and activation are successful, care workers begin to accept individual responsibility for solving problems that their employers have caused, such as understaffing. The logic of self-governance does not change the logic of details, but merely downplays care workers' abilities to object to it. Similarly, middle managers who object and draw public attention to structural problems in their work environment are stigmatised as poor managers who are unable to coach and activate their staff members.

Even if care workers are granted real autonomy and the ability to decide how they organise their daily work, this does not self-evidently help. If the real problem is understaffing and a lack of resources, care workers' increased autonomy does not resolve the problem. In a recent Finnish study, having autonomy in daily work did not decrease care workers' intentions to leave their jobs (Olakivi et al, 2020). In the prevailing management discourse, however, self-governance tends to attract more attention than, for example, understaffing. Self-governance appears as something that middle managers and care workers can (and normatively should) cultivate, while understaffing appears to be out of their control.

The logic of self-governance pressures both care workers and middle managers who become responsible for solving care problems by supporting their subordinates' abilities to govern themselves. The logic of self-governance easily engenders interaction conflicts between care workers and their supervisors – between two female-dominated groups, neither of which are responsible for the prevailing care crises. If a supervisor is responsible for supporting her subordinates' abilities to govern themselves but the subordinates feel that the real problem in care is not their self-governance but the lack of resources, conflicts are likely to emerge (Olakivi, 2018). In a recent survey from Finland, nearly half of care workers in home care felt that their supervisors did not take care workers' concerns about their work overload seriously (Erkkilä, 2018). Middle managers also face contradictory expectations. They are expected to have experience in the care field, to work near the frontline of care work while the major part of their working time is consumed by administrative tasks, financial responsibilities and constant recruitment in order to fill the gaps in their staff caused by high turnover (Antonsson, 2013: 163–165). They are expected to be motivational and inspirational leaders for their subordinates while, in real life, they may have very little working time to support and supervise their staff (Björk et al, 2013: 269; Kröger et al, 2018). Instead of focusing on the (in)actions of business owners, policy-makers and higher-level managers in the field of elder care, the logic of self-governance thus focuses on care workers and their immediate supervisors, and engenders conflicts between them that burden the entire work community (Satka and Hämeenaho, 2015).

The logic of care also applies to care workers and their supervisors, who are in many ways vulnerable and dependent on each other, on their bodies, on social relations in and out of the workplace. These vulnerabilities and dependencies make care workers and their supervisors prone to various unpredictable, situationally changing needs deriving from work but also beyond it, including from family obligations. The argument according to which care organisations can resolve all problems by supporting care workers' self-governance overlooks such needs, vulnerabilities and dependencies (Hoppania et al, 2016). The logic of self-governance merely combines the unpredictability of care with a strong responsibilisation of care workers and their immediate supervisors.

Conclusion

While the deficits and crises in elder care are starker in Finland than in other Nordic countries, the changes managerial reforms as a primary solution to these crises have also been more common than in neighbouring Sweden, for example (see Anttila et al, 2018). The broad ideology of managerialism cannot be reduced to any one type of management. Indeed, critiques of any one style of management often only call for a different, allegedly better style of management, thus reinforcing the ideology of managerialism. This chapter has focused on how two styles of managerial intervention, the more rationalistic logic of details and the predominantly normative logic of self-governance, clash with the logic and rationality of care. The logic of details emphasises the division of care work into specific tasks, the measurement of outputs, and a hierarchical division of labour divided between planning and control on the one hand, and implementation on the other. The logic of self-governance focuses on motivating and activating workers' abilities to control and develop themselves. Common to both management styles is the fact that they overlook care workers' professional and experiential knowledge on care and, at least in the Finnish context, the material circumstances of care provision.

The logic of details constructs a vision of care divided into predefined outputs that are carried out by the care worker with limited participation in the planning of care, and with limited abilities to respond to unpredictable care needs. Here, the care relationship and the logic of care are not the centre of attention. Rather, the focus is on documentable, measurable and manageable outputs of care work. The management of care diverges from care relationships and becomes a field of specialisation for professionals who have expertise in planning and in keeping statistics on care (Kantanen et al, 2015). This development has repercussions for individuals receiving care. While care workers balance between their specified work tasks and clients' wishes, clients have to content themselves with the norms laid down in a system-oriented manner (Andersson et al, 2004).

Unlike the logic of details, which highlights *external* control, the logic of self-governance expects care workers to be *internally* motivated, entrepreneurial, and responsible for implementing good care, for constantly developing themselves, and for being efficient. If the employee fails, the logic of self-governance identifies problems in the worker's values, commitment, responsibility or ability to practise self-governance – and calls for managerial interventions to solve such problems. The task of the manager is to guide the employee in the right direction. The manager has to reassure the care worker that anything is possible with the right attitude – even and especially if this belief conflicts with the employee's experience. Here, as well as in the logic of details, the care worker's knowledge of the work is subjugated to the manager's knowledge. The normative logic of self-governance demands a lot from the manager who, due to their own work overload, may have limited abilities to support their subordinates.

The analysis of different management trends and their combinations from the logic of care perspective responds to the question of why care crises continue to occur even after decades of developing care management. Simply put, care is difficult to manage. While we do not intend to deny that elder care would benefit from good management, our discussion has demonstrated that business-like management models are a poor fit for the realities of care work. Prevailing management styles that are in conflict with the logic and rationality of care can aggravate, not alleviate, care crises. Importantly, the political focus on management easily obscures the root causes of the crisis relating to the under-resourcing and undervaluing of gendered and embodied professional care work. As long as the political focus continues to downplay the fact that care is a labour-intensive sector and that good care can only be achieved with a sufficient number of valued and educated professional workers whose work is organised respecting the logic of care, crises will occur.

References

Adams, T.L. (2010) 'Gender and feminization in health care professions', *Sociology Compass*, 4(7): 454–465.

Ahosola, P. and Lumme-Sandt, K. (2019) 'Vanhustyön kehittämishankkeet vanhuspalvelujärjestelmän vastuita rakentamassa', *Janus*, 27(3): 228–245.

Andersson, S., Haverinen, R. and Malin, M. (2004) 'Vanhusten kotihoito kolmesta näkökulmasta: vanhukset, työntekijät ja johto integroinnin ja asiakaskeskeisyyden arvioijina', *Yhteiskuntapolitiikka*, 69(5): 481–494.

Anttila, T., Oinas, T.S. and Mustosmäki, A. (2018) 'Towards formalisation: The organisation of work in the public and private sectors in Nordic countries', *Acta Sociologica*, 62(3): 315–333.

Anttonen, A. and Zechner, M. (2011) 'Theorizing care and care work' in B. Pfau-Effinger and T. Rostgaard (eds) *Care Between Work and Welfare in European Societies*, Houndmills: Palgrave Macmillan, pp 15–34.

Antonsson, H. (2013) *Chefers arbete i äldreomsorgen – att hantera den svårhanterliga omvärlden. Relationen mellan arbete och organisering*, Linköpig: Linköpings universitet.

Arnkil, R. (2004) 'The Finnish workplace development programme: A small giant?', *Concepts and Transformation*, 9(3): 249–278.

Astvik, W. and Melin, M. (2012) 'Coping with the imbalance between job demands and resources: A study of different coping patterns and implications for health and quality in human service work', *Journal of Social Work*, 13(4): 337–360.

AVI (2020) 'Tiedotteet [bulletins] 2020', Aluehallintovirastot [Regional State Administrative Agencies], Available from: www.avi.fi/web/avi/tiedotteet-2020 [accessed 23 March 2020].

Baines, D., Charlesworth, S., Cunningham, I. and Dassinger, J. (2012) 'Self-monitoring, self-blaming, self-sacrificing workers: Gendered managerialism in the non-profit sector', *Women's Studies International Forum*, 35(5): 362–371.

Banerjee, A. (2013) 'The regulatory trap: Reflections on the vicious circle of regulation in Canadian residential care' in G. Meagher and M. Szebehely (eds) *Marketisation in Nordic Elder care: A Research Report on Legislation, Oversight, Extent and Consequences*, Stockholm: Stockholm University, pp 203–215.

Björk, L., Bejerot, E., Jacobshagen, N. and Härenstam, A. (2013) 'I shouldn't have to do this: Illegitimate tasks as a stressor in relation to organizational control and resource deficits', *Work and Stress*, 27(3): 261–277.

Boltanski, L. and Chiapello, E. (2005) *The New Spirit of Capitalism*, London: Verso.

Bolton, S.C. (2005) '"Making up" managers: The case of NHS nurses', *Work, Employment and Society*, 19(1): 5–23.

Boyd, C. (2002) 'Customer violence and employee health and safety', *Work, Employment and Society*, 16(1): 151–169.

Dahl, H.M. (2009) 'New Public Management, care and struggles about recognition', *Critical Social Policy*, 29(4): 634–654.

Dahl, H.M. (2012) 'Who can be against quality: A new story about home-based care: NPM and governmentality' in C. Ceci, K. Bjørnsdottir and M.E. Purkis (eds) *Perspectives on Care at Home for Older People*, New York: Routledge, pp 139–157.

Diefenbach, T. (2009) 'New Public Management in public sector organizations: The dark side of managerialistic "enlightment"', *Public Administration*, 87(4): 892–909.

Du Gay, P., Salaman, G. and Rees, B. (1996) 'The conduct of management and the management of conduct: Contemporary managerial discourse and the constitution of the "competent" manager', *Journal of Management Studies*, 33(3): 263–282.

Erkkilä, S. (2018) *'Jos tää meno jatkuu, meidän sydämet särkyy': selvitys työstä kotihoidossa ja kotihoitotyön kehittämisestä 2018*, Helsinki: SuPer ry.

Fisher, B. and Tronto, J. (1990) 'Toward a feminist theory of caring' in E.K. Abel and M. Nelson (eds) *Circles of Care*, New York: Albany State University of New York Press, pp 35–62.

Gilbert, T.P. (2005) 'Trust and managerialism: Exploring discourses of care', *Journal of Advanced Nursing*, 52(4): 454–463.

Grey, C. (1999) '"We are all managers now"; "we always were": On the development and demise of management', *Journal of Management Studies*, 36(5): 561–585.

Heikkilä, R., Björkgren, M., Vesa, M., Viitanen, B., Laine, A., Taimi, K., Noro, A., Mäkelä, M., Asikainen, J., Sohlman, B., Hammar, T., Mäkinen, L., Andreasen, P. and Finne-Soveri, H. (2014) *Asiakasryhmittelyyn pohjautuva tuotteistus RUG-III/18-luokituksen avulla. Kotihoito Tampereella*, Helsinki: THL, Available from: www.julkari.fi/bitstream/handle/10024/116771/URN_ISBN_978-952-302-309-3.pdf;jsessionid=29D7054A95 4B7CA193F4D34D6D1263E4?sequence=1 [accessed 25 March 2020].

Henriksson, L. and Wrede, S. (2008) 'Care work in the context of a transforming welfare state' in S. Wrede, L. Henriksson, H. Høst, S. Johansson and B. Dybbroe (eds) *Care Work in Crisis: Reclaiming the Nordic Ethos of Care*, Lund: Studentlitteratur, pp 129–130.

Henriksson, L., Wrede, S. and Burau, V. (2006) 'Understanding professional projects in welfare service work: Revival of old professionalism?', *Gender, Work and Organization*, 13(2): 174–192.

Hirvonen, H. and Husso, M. (2012) 'Hoivatyön ajalliset kehykset ja rytmiristiriidat', *Työelämän tutkimus*, 10(2): 119–133.

Hirvonen, H., Mankki, L., Lehto, I. and Jokinen, E. (2020) 'Ammatillinen toimijuus lean-ajattelussa' in J. Kantola, P. Koskinen Sandberg and H. Ylöstalo (eds) *Tasa-arvopolitiikan suunnanmuutoksia. Talouskriisistä tasa-arvon kriiseihin*, Helsinki: Gaudeamus, pp 234–261.

Hoppania, H.-K. (2015) *Care as a Site for Political Struggle*, publications of the Department of Political and Economic Studies 25, Helsinki: University of Helsinki, Available from: https://helda.helsinki/bitstream/handle/10138/157561/careasas.pdf?sequence=1 [accessed 15 December 2016].

Hoppania, H.-K. and Vaittinen, T. (2015) 'A household full of bodies: Neoliberalism, care and "the political"', *Global Society*, 29(1): 70–88.

Hoppania, H.-K., Olakivi, A. and Zechner, M. (2017) 'Johtamisen rajat vanhushoivassa' in J. Kulmala (ed) *Parempi vanhustyö: menetelmiä johtamisen kehittämiseen*, Jyväskylä: PS-kustannus, pp 202–224.

Hoppania, H.-K., Karsio, O., Näre, L., Olakivi, A., Sointu, L., Vaittinen, T. and Zechner, M. (2016) *Hoivan arvoiset: vaiva yhteiskunnan ytimessä*, Helsinki: Gaudeamus.

Hussein, S., Ismail, M. and Manthorpe, J. (2016) 'Male workers in the female-dominated long-term care sector: Evidence from England', *Journal of Gender Studies*, 25(1): 35–49.

Kantanen, K., Kaunonen, M. and Helminen, M. (2015) 'The development and pilot of an instrument for measuring nurse managers' leadership and management competencies', *Journal of Research in Nursing*, 20(8): 667–677.

Karsio, O. and Anttonen, A. (2013) 'Marketisation of elder care in Finland: Legal frames, outsourcing practices and the rapid growth of for-profit services' in G. Meagher and M. Szebehely (eds) *Marketisation in Nordic Elder care: A Research Report on Legislation, Oversight, Extent and Consequences*, Stockholm: Stockholm University, pp 85–124.

King, D. (2012) 'It's frustrating! Managing emotional dissonance in aged care work', *Australian Journal of Social Issues*, 47(1): 51–70.

Klikauer, T. (2015) 'What is managerialism?', *Critical Sociology*, 41(7–8): 1103–1119.

Kröger, T. (2019) 'Looking for the easy way out: Demographic panic and the twists and turns of long-term care policy in Finland' in T.-K. Jing, S. Kuhnle, Y. Pan and S. Chen (eds) *Aging Welfare and Social Policy*, Cham: Springer, pp 91–104.

Kröger, T., Leinonen, A. and Vuorensyrjä, M. (2009) *Hoivatyön tekijät. Suomalainen hoivatyö pohjoismaisessa tarkastelussa*, Jyväskylä: Jyväskylän yliopisto, Available from: https://jyx.jyu.fi/bitstream/handle/123456789/47699/978-951-39-3691-4.pdf?sequence=1andisAllowed=y [accessed 25 March 2020].

Kröger, T., Puthenparambil, J.M. and Van Aerschot, L. (2019) 'Care poverty: Unmet care needs in a Nordic welfare state', *International Journal of Care and Caring*, 3(4): 485–500.

Kröger, T., Van Aerschot, L. and Puthenparambil, J.M. (2018) *Hoivatyö muutoksessa: suomalainen vanhustyö pohjoismaisessa vertailussa*, YFI julkaisuja, 6, Jyväskylä: Jyväskylän yliopisto, Available from: https://jyx.jyu.fi/bitstream/handle/123456789/57183/978-951-39-7372-8.pdf?sequence=1 [accessed 25 March 2020].

Kurunmaki, L., Mennicken, A. and Miller, P. (2016) 'Quantifying, economising, and marketising: Democratising the social sphere', *Sociologie du Travail*, 58(4): 390–402.

Miller, P. and Rose, N. (2008) *Governing the Present: Administering Economic, Social and Personal Life*, Cambridge: Polity Press.

Moffatt, F., Martin, P. and Timmons, S. (2014) 'Constructing notions of healthcare productivity: The call for a new professionalism?', *Sociology of Health and Illness*, 36(5): 686–702.

Mol, A. (2008) *Logic of Care: Health and the Problem of Patient Choice*, London: Routledge.

Näre, L. (2013) 'Ideal workers and suspects: Employers' politics of recognition and the migrant division of care labour in Finland', *Nordic Journal of Migration Research*, 3(2): 72–81.

Olakivi, A. (2017) 'Unmasking the enterprising nurse: Migrant care workers and the discursive mobilisation of productive professionals', *Sociology of Health and Illness*, 39(3): 428–442.

Olakivi, A. (2018) *The Relational Construction of Occupational Agency: Performing Professional and Enterprising Selves in Diversifying Care Work*, Helsinki: University of Helsinki.

Olakivi, A. (2019) 'The problematic recruitment of migrant labor: A relational perspective on the agency of care work managers', *Current Sociology*, 68(3): 333–352.

Olakivi, A. and Niska, M. (2017) 'Rethinking managerialism in professional work: From competing logics to overlapping discourses', *Journal of Professions and Organization*, 4(1): 20–35.

Olakivi, A., Van Aerschot, L., Puthenparambil, J.M. and Kröger, T. (2020) 'Ylikuormitusta, lähijohtajan tuen puutetta vai vääränlaisia tehtäviä: miksi yhä useammat vanhustyöntekijät harkitsevat työnsä lopettamista?', *Yhteiskuntapolitiikka*, 86(2): 141–154.

Oldenhof, L., Stoopendaal, A. and Putters, K. (2016) 'Professional talk: How middle managers frame care workers as professionals', *Health Care Analysis*, 24(1): 47–70.

O'Reilly, D. and Reed, M. (2010) ' "Leaderism": An evolution of managerialism in UK public service reform', *Public Administration*, 88(4): 960–978.

Paasivaara, L. (2002) 'Tavoitteet ja tosiasiallinen toiminta: suomalaisen vanhusten hoitotyön muotoutuminen monitasotarkastelussa 1930-luvulta 2000-luvulle', Oulu: University of Oulu, Available from: http://jultika. oulu.fi/files/isbn9514269012.pdf [accessed 20 November 2020].

Räsänen, K. and Trux, M.-L. (2012) *Työkirja: ammattilaisen paluu*, Helsinki: Kansanvalistusseura.

Räsänen, R. (2011) *Ikääntyneiden asiakkaiden elämänlaatu ympärivuorokautisessa hoivassa sekä hoivan ja johtamisen laadun merkitys sille*, Acta universitatis Lappoensis 210, Rovaniemi: Lapland University Press, Available from: https://lauda.ulapland.fi/bitstream/handle/10024/61722/R%C3%A4s%C3%A4nen_Riitta_DORIA.pdf?sequence=4 [accessed 24 March 2020].

Satka, M. and Hämeenaho, P. (2015) 'Finnish elder care services in crisis: The viewpoint of rural home care workers', *Nordic Social Work Research*, 5(1): 81–94.

Seppälä, A. (2019) 'Huippututkija: miljardi euroa lisää vuodessa nostaisi Suomen vanhushuollon pohjoismaiselle keskitasolle', *Yle*, 30 January, Available from: https://yle.fi/uutiset/3-10618988 [accessed 24 March 2020].

Sinervo, T., Koponen, E-L., Syrjä, V. and Hietapakka, L. (2013) *Hoiva-avustajaselvitys: joustava koulutus ja työllistymisväylä sosiaali- ja terveyspalveluiden avustaviin tehtäviin*, Helsinki: STM, Available from: http://julkaisut. valtioneuvosto.fi/bitstream/handle/10024/70156/URN_ISBN_978-952-00-3453-5.pdf?sequence=1andisAllowed=y [accessed 25 March 2020].

Sipiläinen, H., Kankkunen, P. and Kvist, T. (2011) 'Kaltoinkohtelu vanhainkodeissa – hoitotyön johtajien käsityksiä altistavista tekijöistä ja ennaltaehkäisystä', *Gerontologia*, 25(1): 15–26.

Sitra (2018) *Ilmiömäinen julkinen hallinto: keskustelualoite valtioneuvoston toimintatapojen uudistamiseksi*, Helsinki: Sitra, Available from: https://media. sitra.fi/2018/09/03163806/ilmiomainenjulkinenhallinto.pdf [accessed 25 March 2020].

Statistics Finland (2019) Labour statistics on foreign-born employees available on request from www.stat.fi.

Stenman, P., Vähäkangas, P., Salo, P., Kivimäki, M. and Paasivaara, L. (2015) 'Henkilöstön työtyytyväisyys vanhustenhuollossa – kohti kuntoutumista edistävän hoitotyön toimintamallin käyttöönottoa', *Hoitotiede*, 27(1): 31–42.

STM (2017) *Laatusuositus hyvän ikääntymisen turvaamiseksi ja palvelujen parantamiseksi 2017–2019*, Sosiaali- ja terveysministeriön julkaisuja 2017:6, Helsinki: Sosiaali- ja terveysministeriö, Available from: http:// julkaisut.valtioneuvosto.fi/bitstream/handle/10024/80132/06_2017_ Laatusuositusjulkaisu_fi_kansilla.pdf?sequence=1andisAllowed=y [accessed 24 March 2020].

Surakka, T., Suonsivu, K. and Åstedt-Kurki, P. (2014) 'Vanhustyön lähijohtajien näkemyksiä hyvästä vanhuksen kanssa tehtävästä työstä', *Gerontologia*, 28(4): 221–230.

THL (2018) 'Vanhuspalvelujen tila', Helsinki: THL, Available from: https:// thl.fi/fi/web/ikaantyminen/muuttuvat-vanhuspalvelut/vanhuspalvelujen-tila [accessed 25 March 2020].

Tiessalo, P. (2019) 'Akuutti kriisi päällä, asiakasturvallisuus vaarassa hoivakoti Ulrikassa – kunta otti toiminnan vastuulleen', *Yle*, 26 January, Available from: https://yle.fi/uutiset/3-10615577 [accessed 20 March 2020].

Trevithick, P. (2014) 'Humanising managerialism: Reclaiming emotional reasoning, intuition, the relationship, and knowledge and skills in social work', *Journal of Social Work Practice*, 28(3): 287–311.

Trydegård, G.-B. (2012) 'Care work in changing welfare states: Nordic care workers' experiences', *European Journal of Ageing*, 9(2): 119–129.

Twigg, J., Wolkowitz, C., Cohen, R.L. and Nettleton, S. (2011) 'Conceptualising body work in health and social care', *Sociology of Health and Illness*, 33(2): 171–188.

Valokivi, H. and Zechner, M. (2009) 'Ristiriitainen omaishoiva – läheisen auttamisesta kunnan palveluksi' in A. Anttonen, H. Valokivi and M. Zechner (eds) *Hoiva – tutkimus, politiikka ja arki*, Tampere: Vastapaino, pp 126–153.

Valvira (2019) 'Vanhustenhoivan epäkohtailmoituksia saatu runsaasti – jokainen otetaan vakavasti', Valvira, 6 March, Available from: www.valvira. fi/-/vanhustenhoivan-epakohtailmoituksia-saatu-runsaasti-jokainen-otetaan-vakavasti [accessed 15 May 2020].

Vehko, T., Sinervo, T. and Josefsson, K. (2017) *Henkilöstön hyvinvointi vanhuspalveluissa — kotihoidon kehitys huolestuttava*, Tutkimuksesta tiiviisti 11, Helsinki: THL, Available from: www.julkari.fi/bitstream/handle/10024/134678/URN_ISBN_978-952-302-876-0.pdf?sequence=1 [accessed 25 March 2020].

Waerness, K. (1984) 'The rationality of caring', *Economic and Industrial Democracy*, 5(2): 185–211.

Yle (2006) 'Tampereelle huomautus hoitajapulasta', *Yle*, 30 March, Available from: https://yle.fi/uutiset/3-5224104 [accessed 6 April 2020].

Zechner, M. (2008) 'Kykyjä kyvyttömyyden tasolla: hoivan vaiheet vanhusten kertomana', *Janus*, 16(4): 295–310.

7

'We are here for you': the care crisis and the (un)learning of good nursing

Carsten Juul Jensen and Steen Baagøe Nielsen

Introduction

Over the last few decades, nurses have had to do the necessary, and sometimes life-saving, care work at hospitals under genuinely changing political and organisational conditions. Following the regimes of New Public Management (NPM), new managerial discourses have been set up in Scandinavia, as well as in many other OECD countries, which have placed ever-increasing pressure on health-care workers (Malmmose, 2009; Centeno and Cohen, 2012). Managerial regimes have been implemented, partly to encourage efficiency through standardisation of care, but also to ensure commitment to the marketisation discourse and make 'health care services' more consumer-oriented and open, to meet the consumer's 'right to choose' between different service providers. The arrival of these new regimes and discourses have been followed by policy instructions to take up a more service-minded approach, displayed through the slogan, 'We are here for you', advertising the Regional Health Service on the website (Region Sjælland, 2016). This is part of a policy regime, aiming to address the needs of patients-as-customers and announcing the political and organisational concern, not only for consumer choices, but also for their safety – as a first priority. While it could in fact be seen as a commitment to address citizens' and patients' needs, we will discuss a different and more complex reality. The focus of this chapter is on the consequences of the current transformations of these governing regimes – here based on the recorded experiences of newly educated nurses from different medical wards in Region Zealand, Denmark.

The work of nurses has, since the beginning of the 21st century, been deeply influenced by international discourses of safety programmes; especially as outlined in the World Health Organisation's (WHO) conceptualisation of 'patient safety friendly hospitals' (WHO, 2016). These safety programmes are clearly linked to the discursive visions of NPM to improve health care services to secure consumer satisfaction, directly targeting the issue of reliability of services. The organisational commitments have led to intensified monitoring of care practices, shifting the implied responsibilities towards the professionals rather than the patients (Mitchel, 2008), which has imposed further demands on health professionals to safeguard patients from the risk of malpractice in the name of patient-centredness.

These discourses have had major impact on the reform of the municipal, regional and state health services in Denmark in 2007, and the slogan 'We are here for you' (Region Sjælland, 2016) can be seen as an example of such impact, with its statement of wholehearted commitment to ensure the care of the patient along with the WHO visions. The Region Zealand's website explains:

> The statement is a commitment, and we do expect to be measured by our efforts. We are ready to be made accountable. The new slogan of Region Zealand should make it clear to everyone we are in contact with, that we wish to create the best imaginable service and quality. (Region Sjælland, 2016)

The message invites every citizen, as 'service consumer', to clearly acknowledge that Region Zealand is a trustworthy 'service provider' of high-quality patient centred treatment. This type of service-minded approach is typical of NPM-led reforms in Denmark, where government financing 'follow patients choices', rather than distributed costs for the particular hospital treatment (Andersen and Jensen, 2010).

Thus, the 'we-are-here-for-you' perspective should be understood as part of broader managerial discourses of consumers' 'right to choose', to attract and make them 'loyal customers'. The imprecise but all-encompassing 'we' of the slogan seems to represent a *corporate body*, which potentially encompasses everyone from the politicians, to management, to 'front-line staff' in the units communicating a message of safety and service-mindedness to the consumer, 'you', that is the citizens/consumers of Region Zealand. The primary pressures, however, are put on the immediate delivery of service – in the direct relationship with the patient, where nurses and other health-care personnel must abide to the slogan and perform accordingly to attract and retain patients through the provision of a quality of care and treatment, delivering 'value for money'.

This chapter's discussion is based on the recorded experiences and practices of newly qualified nurses, how their 'handling' of pressures put them under individualised stress by the reformed hospitals, as well as performative demands following NPM, which led to the reduction of relational, empathetic care practices. The nurses experience a *care squeeze*, in which the individual nurse in her daily practices must learn to do care work either through workarounds and instrumentalisation or by compensating for the reduced and insufficient services through appropriating their own individual, 'private' capacities and qualifications (Rasmussen and Rasmussen, 2012). In the following we discuss particular experiences of newly qualified nurses as both exemplary and indicative of dimensions of a broader 'care crisis' in the context of health care in the reformed public 'patient safety friendly hospitals' of the Nordic welfare state.

Conceptualising a crisis of care and its drain on human capacity and qualifications

Theoretically, we base the discussion on three conceptual inspirations. First, the understandings of practitioners (the newly qualified nurses [NQNs] that are focus in this chapter) as *knowers* of their actual working condition, and *experts* of their everyday activities, work practices and workarounds that are necessary to cope with work pressures imposed by the political, organisational and discursive *'ruling relations'* at work. These concepts have been developed by Dorothy Smith in her conceptualisation of Institutional Ethnography (IE) in line with the Marxist, feminist tradition of standpoint theory (Smith, 2005). Methodologically, this means that we as researchers follow in the footsteps of the practitioners to track how their work and how their everyday knowledge about their work practices are both shaped and reduced by the 'invariable ruling social, political and economic relations' (Smith, 2005). We shall return to unfold these perspectives which have both methodological and theoretical consequences.

Second, we relate these analytical concepts to the broader concepts of *care crisis* and *boundary struggles* developed by Nancy Fraser (2013, 2014, 2016) similarly based on a Marxist feminist approach. We draw on Fraser's theories of 'care crises' and the contemporary radicalisation of *boundary struggles* to stress how the general transformations of care and reproduction relate to the expansion of 'financialised capitalism'. These central concepts capture how the ongoing shifts in central discourses and everyday practices have effects on the transformations of the overall relationship between 'production' and care work (reproductive work), adding to the rising pressure on the human foundations of care. In this way we attempt to point to the ways that the 'ruling relations', described by Smith, are not simply the result of a change in public governance, but are in fact a consequence of growing neoliberal pressures added on the public provision of care.

In her book *Fortunes of Feminism: From State-Managed Capitalism to Neoliberal Crisis* (Fraser, 2013) and subsequent articles (Fraser, 2014, 2016), Fraser argues for the appearance of an extensive crisis following cutbacks in public spending on social and health care services; which, especially since the 1980s, has led to a drain on care capacity. This has transformed the terms and possibilities of public health care. Fraser points to the fundamental and contradictory dynamics of capital accumulation, which serves to undermine the 'social reproduction' – of which care work is of course a central part – in order to maximise profits: 'capitalism's orientation to unlimited accumulation tends to destabilise the very processes of social reproduction on which it relies' (Fraser, 2016: 100).

Fraser explores this neoliberal process of undermining and destabilisation through a historical analysis of the transformation of care work in three 'regimes of accumulation' where 'production has assumed a different institutional form', namely: (1) *Housewifisation* – and domestication of care (from the 19th century), whereby women's labour simply becomes considered 'a natural resource'; (2) *State-managed capitalism* (of the 20th century), which 'internalized social reproduction through state and corporate provision of social welfare'; and (3) the present regime of *Financialised capitalism*. This regime is internationally characterised by a 'diminishing public provision, and radical (re)privatisation of care work' (Fraser, 2016: 104). In this chapter we discuss the difficulties of the approaching third regime – especially as they appear in the Nordic context where the institutionalisation of the second regime seems to have been partly resistant to the most extensive wave of privatisation.

Third, care researchers in the Nordic countries have contributed with contextual analyses and conceptualisations of the ways that care workers (predominantly women) have reacted to the dismantling of the 'second regime'; that is, the 'reorganisation' and partial privatisation of the hitherto very well-established public provision of social and health care services (Wrede et al, 2008; Dahl et al, 2011; Kamp and Hvid, 2012). Nordic care researchers have shown on the one side how this 'second regime' has been particularly developed in the Nordic countries, with extensive public funding and institutionalisation. They have pointed to the ways care workers have been able to maintain a high quality of care, based on a well-educated (bachelor's degree) staff of care workers; despite the fact that neoliberal, financialised political pressure has put this 'regime' under threat with attempts to rationalise, privatise and marketise health-care services. The Nordic countries, however, may be said to have seen a less radical institutional dismantling of publicly organised services than the one recorded in Anglo-American research.[1] Such research shows how NPM-led reform of public hospitals has, especially since the start of the 21st century, involved the introduction of private sector management models and governing regimes to the administrations of hospitals. This was followed by policies and governance to control and implement formal measures for quality assurance – directly linked to economic performance and the idea of 'value for money' (Rasmussen and Rasmussen, 2012). Today, it becomes still more apparent that care work in the Nordic countries, despite remaining predominantly publicly funded and organised, is still exposed to *boundary struggles* around the possibilities of a strong future for a publicly financed health sector. The boundary struggle here concerns the intensified expropriation of (mainly women's) individual abilities and willingness to care, and the continued undermining of basic material and human conditions through the (re)organisation of care work within the public sector. (Rasmussen and Rasmussen, 2012; Fraser, 2014, 2016). In order to track the specific difficulties in the daily practices of care work, we will supplement the understanding of care crisis with concepts of a *care squeeze* (Dahl et al, 2011), which we use here to capture the practical experience of the undermining of (pre)condition and standards of care, also in the context of Nordic NPM-led 'modernisation' programmes of the public sector services and the neo-liberal call for 'value for money'. (Wrede et al, 2008; Kamp and Hvid, 2012).

'Modernisation' of Nordic public services: 'value for money'

Consequences relating to the two 'ends' of the 'value for money' ideals of the new governing regime in the health sector have been twofold: first, a generally slow but continued cut back in the 'money', that is, the economic budgets of hospitals. Second, a new political focus on improved 'value', as measured through the legitimacy and reputation of the services, with the intended aim of holding on to 'customers' and improving their experience of quality. As we discussed earlier, the discursive focus on 'modernising' through underlining both safety and patient-orientation goes hand-in-hand with a basic strategy of marketisation of services – as expressed in the slogan 'We are here for you'. Though, part of this strategy also stresses the qualitative 'value'-dimensions of these services, the understanding of 'value' is of course somewhat vague and illusive at least from the perspective of governance. Therefore a lot of effort has been put into creating accountability and performance measures (Christiansen and Vrangbæk, 2018). However, the discourses of 'value', 'quality', 'patient-centredness' and 'safety' all have the immediate effect of reframing the caring practices in such a way that they seem to put the service-orientation and patient-centred care first. These ideals are further promoted through the Danish accreditation for health-care providers (DKKM) with national goals for patient safety and service standards imposed through separate governing bodies (IKAS, 2012).

There is however a downside to this priority, as emphasised by the governing bodies: the politically determined national goals are considered, in formal evaluations of the administrative costs of DKKM, as being set too high compared to a reasonable outcome of patient safety – despite the fact that the goals are (still) not met according to continuous measurements (Holm-Petersen and Højgaard, 2018). As a result, the managerial focus of these 'patient safety friendly hospitals' (WHO, 2016) has been directed towards economically driven incentives to secure 'workforce efficiency' from the health service's professional staff (Holm–Petersen and Højgaard, 2018). This shift towards the fiscal end of the 'value for money' equation has in Denmark instigated a series of politically driven organisational reforms for the termination of 20 per cent of the emergency units, and a general demand to increase hospital productivity by 2 per cent per year (Christiansen, 2012). These budget cuts that went on for years, have, of course, had real consequences for the working conditions; not least in the medical units where patients are often senior citizens (over 80 years old), hospitalised with acute illnesses that require intensive specialised treatment in 80 per cent of cases (Hansen, 2014). Such patients often have multifactorial and complex diseases and remain in care for longer periods – for example, five days, compared to the overall average of two days. This group of patients has increased in number by 71 per cent from 1980 to 2016 (Danmarks Statistik, 2016). The budget cuts have also caused an increased workload pressure on hospital staff. The Danish Nurses' Organisation states that 38 per cent of hospital nurses report that busyness can affect patient safety negatively due to understaffing (DSR, 2019). This reflects another international trend, the focus on rationalisation and financial cutbacks, which has demanded that the workforce work more efficiently (Rankin and Campbell, 2006).

'Modernisation' discourses undermine nurses' educational competence

The practical understanding of good patient–centred care is originally based on well-established discourses and conceptualisations of 'ethical standards' drawing upon pillars of nursing education taught to generations of nurses and other health professionals. Though the union of nurses has over the last decades attempted to follow a strategy of professionalisation to secure and further develop the qualities of the 'second regime' of publicly funded health care. This project relies on the traditional image of nursing and its ethical standards, which still feeds into the traditional recruitment of nurses among young dedicated women (Eriksen, 2004). The somewhat idealized obligation of nurses, according to the ethical standards, has always been to put the patient's need first, to meet patients and peers with a pleasant, kind, self-sacrificing and caring 'femininity', so that the individual patient feels comfortable, no matter the working conditions of the staff themselves (Martinsen, 2010). The common educational discourse of the 'good nurse' taught at nursing colleges draws heavily on the writings of Martinsen (2010), where nurses' behaviour seem to naturally conform to norms of sympathy for suffering patients, that is, compassionate care. These basically humanistic ideals and ethical standards draw upon the ideology of traditional pastoral powers, taught to generations of nurses following in the footsteps of Florence Nightingale, and her naturalising credo: *every woman is a nurse* (Gordon and Nelson, 2005), that nursing practices must be performed on the (gendered) 'personal moral fibre' of the supposedly selfless (female) nurse. Although parts of the nurses' professional project linked to the 'second regime' has been pursued on the basis of a stronger trust and commitment to practical clinical knowledge, and a knowledge base closer to the bio-medical and natural sciences, the humanistic understanding of care is still considered fundamental – especially in areas where the prospects of medical 'cure' is often overshadowed by the need for (often even terminal) care (Eriksen, 2004).

As we have discussed, nursing of the 21st century has been undergoing significant changes following redefined managerial regimes, new organisational structures and the discourses of NPM. Nurses must, to a wide extent, adapt to new structures of work, as they will otherwise be labelled institutionally as outmoded, incapable, rigid or as slow workers (Rankin and Campbell, 2006; Jensen, 2018). This of course calls for some revisions in the current narrative of nursing (Rankin and Campbell, 2006), however, most nurses especially within the medical units still proclaim the need for a sturdy and resilient approach to patients, and as a result will often experience 'care squeeze' (Jensen, 2018).

In the following analysis we discuss the consequences of care crisis and care squeeze by contextualising experiences using new empirical material from Danish hospital units.

Method and design

The empirical work of the chapter was undertaken as part of a PhD fellowship (Jensen, 2018), based on the IE methods of Smith (2005). The basic understanding here is that the participants as NQNs are understood to possess *local expert knowledge* on their everyday practice at the medical units. The analysis draws on the principles of IE, with its attempt to be procedural and descriptive, based on the everyday experiences of the nurses who participated (DeVault and McCoy, 2006; Rankin, 2017). Although the NQNs' actual practices are essential, the recordings and description of practices also serve to uncover the influences of discourses and other ruling relations of the institution.

By tracking the use of practices and the importance they are given in central documents of the institution, the ethnographer can detect the workings of discourses supporting the ruling relations that frame the institutional activities. From this, one may track the different (even subversive) identification of actors' problems, or as Smith insists of everyday life people, as they are put under pressure (Smith, 2005).

Discourses and other ruling relations create tensions and discrepancies – generally leading to the reproduction of these ruling relations. Actors may feel alienated, but they will respond – do, think and feel – and often make *workarounds* to meet these ruling relations (Smith, 2005). Hence, by following and analysing the activities and experiences of NQNs in medical units from their standpoint, it enables us to understand the nurses' appropriation of, and responses to, the central discourses; and additionally, the way these discourses work to create certain forms of work knowledge and eliminate or marginalise other forms of knowledge (Rankin and Campbell, 2006).

Data collection took place over a 184-hour period, in four medical units, at one hospital in Region Zealand, Denmark. The four units routinely hire NQNs during their first two weeks immediately after graduation, of which, three NQNs (Emilie, Rebecca, Anja – here named with pseudonyms) are cited in this chapter. Moreover, the ethnography also followed 20 health professionals (nurses and auxiliaries) in their everyday (and every-night) work life from 1 June 2015 to late October 2016.

Observations were complemented with multiple ethnographic interviews, open-ended dialogues in hospital meeting rooms, private homes, cafés, or by telephone. Further follow-ups were by personal semi-structured interviews, through which the NQNs and other participants were asked about their practices and motivations, from a starting point of observed work situations over a period of all together 18 months. Moreover, the analysis is based on a reading of corporate texts in order to reach beyond the immediately observable data of participant observation and personal interviews (Jensen, 2018). We have thus analysed documents related to patient safety in Denmark (Danish Patient Safety Authority, n.d.; Ministeriet for Sundhed og Forebyggelse, 2014; Danske regioner, 2015; Ministry of Health, 2016; Region Sjælland, 2016) to map the 'ruling relations' of the organisation.

In the following vignettes of the nurses' work life in the medical units, we show a range of responses to politically determined workload pressure on hospital staff following budget cuts and performative demands. Through these vignettes we aim to add empirical depth to Fraser's understanding of care crises, as it takes the form of pressures in the lives of NQNs.

Tracing nurses' experiences of health system discourses and economic rationalisation

Emilie: care under pressure

The first vignette follows Emilie at a regional medical hospital unit in Denmark:

At 8 am, I [Jensen – author] followed Emilie. She was stuck in a ward to help a patient who had wet himself. She patiently helped him to wash his body and change his clothes, with a gentle facial expression.

On our way out, afterwards, she reflected in the corridor: 'I get so frustrated when I cannot keep my promises. I forgot to ask someone [another patient] about breakfast, and I know, there was another patient we had to help with the food'.

Here, Emilie provides practical, gentle care for the patient who had wet himself. Though Emilie's actions seemed not only fair and necessary, and her priorities are typical of everyday nursing, she was at the same time frustrated being unable to help another patient with breakfast, as she – in her opinion – had broken her promises. Although she had no chance of predicting or handling the patient's urination in any different manner, Emilie explains that she feels guilt as she – in her own opinion – has not been able to respond in a satisfactory way and accommodate both the needs of the patients and colleagues' expectations. As a consequence, Emilie blamed herself. She felt obliged to state that keeping promises is a core value to her, and that she has failed, though such "interruptions" are absolutely unavoidable and impossible to predict. Although "breaking promises" is unavoidable, Emilie's self-esteem was further harmed as she confessed that she imagined that her colleagues would think disparagingly of her as an "unprofessional nurse". Being an NQN, her frustrations were not only related to her own practices but were interpreted in the light of her practical learning process to adapt to the working conditions – and a fear that her reputation would be harmed. During a follow-up interview, she thus reflected: "Then I wonder if my colleagues think, 'What kind of training has she had? She doesn't know a thing!'"

Here, the nurse reflects in recognisable ways over the experienced consequences of common time pressures. Emilie's considerations take a starting point in her expectations to be able to accommodate to 'her' patient's needs, without involving colleagues. Based on the traditional ethics of selfless, good nursing, she feels uncomfortable asking a colleague for help, worried that she/he will be occupied with assisting patients themselves. Despite Emilie's engagement in individualised selfless care, she still blames herself, asking questions and expressing doubts about her abilities and the quality of her education – implicitly taking for granted that her colleagues should be able to do what obviously cannot be done: to be with two patients at the same time, or guard yourself against unexpected incidences.

Rebecca: dismantling the basic rationales of nursing

The discrepancies between the realities of the workload and the discourses of selflessness in the 'patient safety friendly hospital' creates a care squeeze, challenging the whole idea of 'value for money'. The common experience of understaffing is illustrated in Rebecca's experiences at work, two weeks after she had been employed:

Rebecca described an event on a night shift that made her blame herself for taking the wrong decision when a patient died. At 7 am, a couple of bells were ringing from the bathrooms. One of the two nurses on duty (the other), was in the process of reporting on the night's incidental problems to nursing staff that had just met on day shift. Rebecca and the other nurse had 15 minutes – between 7:00 and 7:15 am – to report any problems and issues around the 24 patients present on the ward. Rebecca had her colleague report on 'her' 12 patients, so she was the only one to answer both patients' bells. The first patient proved time-consuming, and therefore it took Rebecca quite a while before she could go and 'answer' the call of the second bell. When entering this second ward she had a shock: 'I opened the door and couldn't see anyone until I noticed the legs of a woman wrapped up in the clothes rack. Her face was blue'. Rebecca found this patient, who unexpectedly had collapsed from acute dyspnoea [breathing difficulties] into the clothes rack. Resuscitation was unsuccessful and Rebecca reflected, 'Why did I do bathroom 6 first?'

Rebecca did indeed provide care as best she could, however her efforts and random choice of ward led to fatal loss of the patient's life – the patient died. Despite her legitimate attempts to meet the hospital regimes, and resuscitate the patient, she blamed herself afterwards for her potentially fatal decision. She seemed to reflect that, if she had chosen to answer the other bell, resuscitation could have been initiated earlier, which might have saved the patient. Moreover, Rebecca did not demand improved working conditions, better support from colleagues or fewer patients. Instead, she blamed herself for making a wrong choice, even if she found it a little strange that the ward nurses sent her home (Rebecca could not be offered overtime pay), as she was the one who knew the patient. The experience made her feel unhappy and annoyed, but still Rebecca did not talk to any staff nurses about the overwhelming experience of the previous morning. Instead, as she recounted during an interview: "It was upsetting, but I could talk to my boyfriend about it." The conversation took place during a night shift, with just her boyfriend present. She stated:

'It helped talking about it the next day with a nurse who was there too. We went in and looked at the computer. The nurse I spoke to also said: 'If only I'd noticed that she had a high pulse rate yesterday!' but then she reminded herself something like: "Yeah, well, but that's the case for half the patients in this ward". So I keep believing that she suffered from a pulmonary embolism [blockage of an artery in the lungs]. You'd have to keep on believing it'.

The experienced nurse seemed to want to teach Rebecca that it is above human capacity to predict or avoid death or cardiac arrest; the cause was indeterminable and could have originated from a general state of acute dyspnoea or critical illness of elderly medical patients, who usually have poor blood circulation in conjunction with a high pulse rate.

Thus, the health system discourse of good patient–centred nursing feeds into the practical handling of the politically determined goals of patient safety programmes set up to rescue patients. Clinicians and management are obliged to monitor patients, but work conditions and demands do in fact not allow for this. Perhaps, the death of Rebecca's patient could have been avoided if Rebecca had not been forced to choose which patient to care for. Rebecca's self-blaming attitude is therefore fully understandable; however, in her eyes, the stressful event was solely due to her inability to make a correct judgement – or work (even) faster. The goals and expected practices of patient safety programmes to a certain extent, rely on or exploit Rebecca's dedication to her work – and in a way seem to work to "translate" her perceived "lack of ability" as a means to make the care system as such seem to appear functional despite its obvious institutional limitations.

Anja: squeezed between 'everyday nursing practice' and 'patient safety-friendly hospitals'

By following Anja, we gained further insights to the difficulties of meeting the contradictory demands of patient-centredness requiring further selflessness, exposing the working of the ruling relations behind them:

> At 7.30 am, after the morning report, I [Jensen] overheard a conversation where an experienced nurse said to Anja as she was leaving the nurses' office, 'I didn't talk much to 11.2. [indicating number of ward and bed of patient] yesterday, I think I'd better give him some care today'. During observations, Anja seemed quite familiar with this nurse after one and a half months working together, and she responded with a wry smile: 'Now you sound like a nursing philosopher'. The experienced nurse hesitated a moment before they laughed together, and then went off to patient number 11.2.

It is obvious from Anja's wry smile that she intended to be ironic, hoping to amuse her colleague. The ironic statement and following laughter might suggest that Anja felt confidence in using irony, which could indicate a certain strength and emotional reserve to engage in informal interactions with her colleague after only six weeks' work experience. However, it could also express resonance, acceptance or even empathy between

Anja and her colleague. Anja's ironic statement indicates an emotional reservation towards her practice, but also an attempt to build a mutually resonant relationship between two colleagues. Anja seemed intentionally to choose ambiguous words that suggest irony and call for some humorous relief (Lynch, 2009).

It seems fair to interpret Anja's response as a type of acceptance of the state of affairs, which also rests on a level of self-defence – confronting the (im)possibilities of ideal care practice. Her indirect reference to the nursing philosopher Martinsen's textbook, *Philosophy of Care* (2010), may be seen as a way of dealing with the care squeeze, and thus an expression of resistance against the institutionally determined working conditions in the medical unit. The reference reminds every nurse of a quite different commonly accepted standard, where fulfilment of patient need is the explicit goal. By reminding her colleague to abstain from the idealism of patient–centred care, Anja not only shows her knowledge of the need to abide to the current standards and working conditions, she also exposes her (perhaps dubious) need to unlearn what she has been taught and emotionally distance herself – and exclude the possibility of making (well-grounded) philosophical reflections about the event.

Conforming to management's customer-oriented 'total quality' discourses

We suggest that the depicted experiences in the vignettes illustrate the nurses' responses to the politically determined workload pressure put on hospital staff. The three nurses respond individually: Anja resort to 'amusing' remarks around the impossibilities of doing patient-centred care according to her (ideal) requirements established during her nursing education. Likewise, Emilie's and Rebecca's (impossible) attempts to fulfil all patients' needs against the organisational realities could be interpreted as the obvious result of an institutionalised policy (and ruling relation), that draws on self-governing principles of nursing practice, exposing them to experiences of inadequacy. As a consequence, it leads the nurses to an individualised self-blame.

Service declarations, such as 'We are here for you', which stress the demands of patients, only add to the performative pressures put on Emilie, Rebecca and, to some extent, Anja. The point here is that the selfless, patient-centred approach that they hold to is far from their own invention or inclination. It is constituted through the discourse of patient–centredness,[2] exposed in the hospital slogan and readily seen on posters in the hallway of the four medical units, on the hospital website, and circulated on every hospital document (Region Sjælland, 2016).

This performative service approach, epitomised in the slogan, was accentuated to the NQNs during their very first introductory seminar for new employees. Here, the hospital manager emphasised the approach: "At our hospital we provide patient-centred care – the mission is the patient and the vision is sovereign – quality isn't just second best, it's total quality." The manager authoritatively stated that patient-centred care should be the best and the overall mission, a declaration to succeed. The manager seemed to realise the dubious implications of the discourse selflessness/patient-centredness in her emphasis during the introduction seminar. In a personal interview, she expressed ambiguity regarding governmental structures: "That's just the way it is, when you need to manoeuvre in political systems. You just have to pick what's most suitable, and if something's crazy, you must figure out what to do with it." To Emilie, Rebecca and Anja, this is much more than 'manoeuvres' or empty (or political) slogans. Such discourses resonate with standards which are traditionally engrained in the health-care system in general and within nurses' professional ethics. Indeed, these standards seem to work performatively.

Some months later, in an interview, Emilie recalled her response when she needed to deliver a handover report (to the evening shift staff).

> 'It had been incredibly busy and there were lots of things I hadn't had time to do. The evening shift staff were talking about how they always had to take over lots of stuff from the day shift. I got so upset. Finished the writing in a hurry and went down to the basement. There I broke down completely.'

Again, Emilie's response exposes how she feels personally responsible for leaving unfinished work for the nurses on the evening shift. This overwhelming frustration, however, does not really correspond in any reasonable way with the common and recurrent experiences on the wards. The sudden pressures from patients' acute needs makes it impossible to overcome all prescribed tasks. Though the nurses from the evening shift might complain slightly, it is hardly likely that anybody would blame Emilie's practice in particular, and thus to an outsider there is in fact little reason for Emilie's experience of insufficiency. For an insider and a 'knower', however, Emilie's reaction is common and, to a certain degree, both expected and necessary.

Conclusion

Data from the underlying institutional ethnography (Jensen, 2018), which we have here only seen examples from, suggest thorough links between the implementation of NPM regimes, new discourses of patient-centredness, and the experience of *care squeeze* felt by the individual nurse – leading to afflicted sufferings.

This adds to previous analyses of a more general 'crisis of care work' in the Nordic countries (Wrede et al, 2008). It offers a deeper understanding of the ways that these discourses draw heavily on the individual abilities of the nurses, as it does not only challenge the educational qualifications of the nurses, but also draws on their individual dedication, as well as their, often private, care experiences and capabilities. This dimension could add to our understanding of the care crises, as it indicates new boundary struggles and the ways that regimes and discourses of care undermine both traditional and more established professional competencies for care.

By accepting the standpoint and knowledge of the nurses around their everyday practices as a starting point, we can show more clearly the ways in which the experienced staff do not only 'live with' the neglect of personal needs. The experienced staff are also eager to show the NQNs that their practices and qualifications acquired from nursing education are in fact idealistic and inappropriate, if one is to remain and 'survive' on the wards. They implicitly, and sometimes even explicitly, stress that 'to be able to work here' – under the given conditions – and maintain the idea that patients' basic needs are actually in focus – vis-à-vis the slogan: 'We are here for you', you need to unlearn what you have been taught.

To overcome the care squeeze, which these situations so clearly demonstrate, workarounds are needed to attempt to provide adaptations to the regular demands and acute situations of day, evening and night shifts, as well as collaboration with colleagues and/or patients with individual, personal characteristics (Rankin and Campbell, 2006). In order to do this, NQNs seem to draw from notions and understandings of selflessness; traditionally valued and sustained in and through their educational training and the (still) dominant professional and idealistic virtues of nursing (which are now fully exploited).

We have here attempted to illustrate the ways the nurses' emotional, 'private' capabilities become invested during their care work. Following how they act as 'knowers', we can acknowledge the way they strive to compensate for the obvious consequences of economic cutbacks and performative discursive pressures of 'patient-centered' care. We see how this comes at a high price. When the newly qualified nurses strive to make up for the poor working conditions in the medical units, their effort to perform 'good nursing' demands an extraordinary effort, which leads to individualised, emotional stress and burn-out, even though their nursing education might have laid a sound foundation for their practice.

In the previous study (Jensen, 2018), two out of five NQNs, of whom four are women, had an emotional breakdown within the first year of their practice. Only one of the five, Thor, seemed to thrive at his new workplace. We cannot here pursue a thorough gendered analysis of these pressures and gendered strategies of coping with the performative pressures of care work.

However, it seems fair to point to the common experience: that male staff in female-dominated care work have a much easier time adapting to the practical conditions of work than the (newly qualified) female nurses and other care workers (Baagøe Nielsen, 2011). While most of the female staff are concerned about the care squeeze, Thor's primary worries are not related to the contents of his job but revolve around his ability to provide for his family; for example, the size of his salary, his ability to buy a house, and what his wife and three children might demand of him. As such, he clings to notions of 'hegemonic masculinity', which seem to 'help' him adapt to a more distanced, 'realistic' approach to care needs. Being less concerned with blame and guilt is commonly seen among fathers (Baagøe Nielsen and Westerling, 2014).

The female nurses, on the other hand, impose on themselves an emotional stress, caused by another kind of 'realism', linked to their attempts to provide patient-centred care. They experience their lack of capacity by failing to meet the needs of the patients, for instance through their lack of ability to predict the urgent and unpredictable needs of acute and critically ill patients, though this would be beyond normal human capacity.

The idealistic understandings of good nursing, which remain active in both education and practice, still rest heavily on feminine connotations, commonly reproduced when journalists describe a nurse as 'a special person, an angel' (Gordon and Nelson, 2006: 25), exposed in the educational literature focusing on nurses' capacity for compassionate patient-centred care (Martinsen, 2010). These understandings, and the professional traditions they go along with, now show themselves 'useful' if the practitioners are indeed encouraged to follow the (performative) idea of patient-centred care, paraphrased in the slogan of Region Zealand: 'We are here for you' (Region Sjælland, 2016), and the foundational understanding of the 'patient safety friendly hospitals' (WHO, 2016).

It is important to point to the organisational and broader social and political framing as contributing to the problems at hand. The costs of policy regimes such as NPM are most often met by neglecting the human resources, the actual skills and the actual knowledge to meet the underlying requirements.

The overall aim of this chapter is to show and discuss the care crisis as it appears in the everyday lives and work of a group of NQNs. Hereby we show how the ruling relations of NPM force the nurses, almost as a rule, to abandon established educational practices and common understandings of good care. The true cost of the care crisis thus appears when the NQNs must challenge their experience of the care squeeze and make workarounds to meet the contradictory demands and pressures related to the changing material and organisational conditions As we have shown this results in breakdown of nurses, and the suffering and even perhaps even premature deaths of patients. When the nurses strive to compensate or limit the dangers of insufficient care, this can, in Fraser's terms, be understood as the result of new boundary struggles. The NQN can from this perspective be seen as the frontline of attempts to transgress prior established boundaries between market (production) and caring (as re-productive institutions). In order to provide proper care for people, who, seen from the perspective of capitalism, are 'non-productive', the nurses must themselves challenge their sense of humanity, as well as their own well-being, to compensate for the incapacities of the organisation. In Fraser's understanding this can be seen as a re-privatisation of care, which she sees directly linked to the current expansion of financialised capitalism.

The boundary struggles come at a high cost, not only for the patients who could have received better care and perhaps even survived the 'adverse events' of the standardised care, but for the NQNs themselves, and this is indeed both frustrating and dramatic. The work itself becomes ingrained with paradoxes and ambivalences that the nurses must individually attempt to alleviate to protect the patients, their families, as well as their own colleagues from the impact of the crisis. As a consequence the NQN must learn to manage their emotions to avoid breakdowns and self-blame. In this way the breakdowns and self-blame of the nurses can be seen as a direct result of the intensified societal and institutional discourses, linked to the overall pressures of the neoliberal regime imposed on the public provision of care.

As such, the experiences of these NQNs expose results of an extensive boundary struggle related to the dismantling of the public care services. This is clearly linked to the ongoing shift in central perceptions of, and discourses around, the relationship between production and care (reproductive work), as well as continued budget cuts, which in fact undermine publicly organised care. This has imposed a shift in focus of the nurses' practices, where the individual nurse can attempt to draw on the humane foundations and ideals of care, solidarity and mutual responsibility in order to oppose regimes working to to undermine established foundations of good nursing. The individual nurse must in fact 'learn' to care differently in order to survive (perhaps one could say in 'traditional masculine ways' – which is a contradiction in terms). They must adapt to 'realistic' modes of care work on the given terms of '(re) production', and '(un)learn' not to use their caring capacities – while at the same time pretend that they are in fact 'here for us'.

Notes

[1] This might seem less apparent in Denmark where the goals of marketisation and privatisation reforms have not been as sweeping as in, for example, the UK, Australia or Latin American countries. Nevertheless, the struggles have worked, in so far as the reforms have had the purpose of creating a new consensus around the legitimacy of a clearly reduced-but-efficient public sector, through the

creation of a public image of delivering 'value-for-money' (Holm-Petersen and Højgaard, 2018).

[2] The understanding of patient-centredness should not be seen as directly synonymous with the popular clinical concept of 'person-centred' care (PCC), though the care orientation in PCC with its ideals of 'shared decision making' in which patients are considered as 'partners' in the design and delivery of services (Gabutti et al, 2017) can be seen as an(other) example of NPMs service-oriented discourses. Current hospital practices seem unable to meet the holistic approach indicated in PCC, and the people in need of care are in fact still considered as patients in a medical sense.

References

Andersen, P.T. and Jensen, J.J. (2010) 'Healthcare reform in Denmark', *Scandinavian Journal of Public Health*, 38(3), 246–252.

Baagøe Nielsen, S. (ed) (2011) *Nordiske mænd til omsorgsarbejde!* København: København: VELPRO – Center for Velfærd, Profession og Hverdagsliv.

Baagøe Nielsen, S. and Westerling, A. (2014) 'Fathering as a learning process: Breaking new grounds in familiar territory' in G.B. Eydal and T. Rostgaard (eds) *Childhood, Youth and Family Life Research*, Bristol: Policy Press, pp 187–208.

Centeno, M.A. and Cohen, J.N. (2012) 'The arc of neoliberalism', *Annual Review of Sociology*, 38(1), 317–340.

Christiansen, T. (2012) 'Ten years of structural reforms in Danish healthcare', *Health Policy*, 106(2), 114–119.

Christiansen, T. and Vrangbæk, K. (2018) 'Hospital centralization and performance in Denmark: Ten years on', *Health Policy*, 122(4), 321–328.

Dahl, H.M., Keränen, M. and Kovalainen, A. (2011) *Europeanization, Care and Gender: Global Complexities*, Basingstoke: Palgrave Macmillan.

Danish Patient Safety Authority (n.d.) *Danish Patient Safety Authority, Homepage*. Available from: https://stps.dk/en

Danmarks Statistik (2016) *Statistisk årbog*, København: Danmarks Statistik.

Danske regioner (Danish Regions) (2015) 'Aftale om regionernes økonomi for 2016', *Danske Regioner (Danish Regions)*. [online] 22 November, Available from: http://www.regioner.dk/aktuelt/nyheder/2015/august/aftale+om+regionernes+-oe-konomi+for+2016 [accessed 29 June 2021].

DeVault, M.L. and McCoy, L. (2006) 'Institutional ethnography: Using interviews to investigate ruling relations' in D.E. Smith (ed) *Institutional Ethnography as Practice*, Lanham, New York, Toronto and Oxford: Rowman & Littlefield, pp 15–44.

DSR (2019) 'NOTAT Sygeplejerskers oplevelse og underbemanding', *DSR analyse/MEGAFON*.

Eriksen, T.R. (2004) 'Gendered professional identity and professional knowledge in female health education: Put into perspective by a follow-up study (1987–2002)', *NORA*, 12(1), 20–30.

Fraser, N. (2013) *Fortunes of Feminism: From State-Managed Capitalism to Neoliberal Crisis*, London and New York: Verso.

Fraser, N. (2014) 'Behind Marx's hidden abode: For an expanded conception of capitalism', *New Left Review*, 86, 55–72.

Fraser, N. (2016) 'Contradictions of capital and care', *New Left Review*, 100(July/August), 99–117.

Gabutti, I., Mascia, D. and Cicchetti, A. (2017) 'Exploring "patient-centered" hospitals: A systematic review to understand change', *BMC Health Services Research*, 17(364), 1–16.

Gordon, S. and Nelson, S. (2005) 'An end to angels', *American Journal of Nursing*, 105(5), 62–69.

Gordon, S. and Nelson, S. (2006) 'Moving beyond the virtue script in nursing' in S. Nelson and S. Gordon (eds) *The Complexities of Care: Nursing Reconsidered*, Ithaca and London: Cornell University Press, pp 13–29.

Hansen, B.V. (2014) *Acute Admissions to Internal Medicine Departments in Denmark: Studies on Admission Rate, Diagnosis, and Prognosis*, PhD dissertation, Department of Clinical Epidemiology, Aarhus University Hospital, Aarhus University.

Holm-Petersen, C. and Højgaard, B. (2018) *Højere kvalitet gennem samling af komplekse og specialiserede kliniske funktioner*, København: Det Nationale Forsknings- og Analysecenter for Velfærd.

IKAS (2012) 'Accreditation standards for hospitals, 2nd version'. [online] 22 November, Available from: http://www.ikas.dk/FTP/PDF/D12-10072.pdf [accessed 29 June 2021].

Jensen, C.J. (2018) *Nyuddannede sygeplejerskers møder med realiteterne på medicinske afsnit i reformerede sygehuse: en institutionel etnografisk undersøgelse*, PhD dissertation, Mennesker og Teknologi, Roskilde Universitet.

Kamp, A. and Hvid, H. (eds) (2012) *Elder care in Transition: Management, Meaning and Identity at Work: A Scandinavian Perspective*, Frederiksberg: Copenhagen Business School Press.

Lynch, O.H. (2009) 'Kitchen antics: The importance of humor and maintaining professionalism at work', *Journal of Applied Communication Research*, 37(4), 444–464.

Malmmose, M. (2009) *New Public Management in Health Care: Its Effects and Implications*, PhD dissertation, Aarhus School of Business, Aarhus University.

Martinsen, K. (2010) *Øjet og Kaldet*. København: Munksgaard.

Ministeriet for Sundhed og Forebyggelse (Health Ministry) (2019) 'Bekendtgørelse af sundhedsloven', *Bekendgørelse (Act of Health)*. Available from: https://www.retsinformation.dk/Forms/r0710.aspx?id=152710 [accessed 29 June 2021]

Ministry of Health (2016) Healthcare in Denmark, AN Overview. Available at: https://www.healthcaredenmark.dk/media/ykedbhsl/healthcare-dk.pdf [accessed 29 June 2021].

Mitchel, P. (2008) 'Patient safety and quality' in R.G. Hughes (ed) *Patient Safety and Quality: An Evidence-Based Handbook for Nurses*, Rockville: Agency for Healthcare Research and Quality, pp 1–5.

Rankin, J. (2017) 'Conducting analysis in institutional ethnography', *International Journal of Qualitative Methods*, 16(1), 1–11.

Rankin, J. and Campbell, M. (2006) *Managing to Nurse Inside Canada's Health Care Reform*, Toronto, Buffalo and London: University of Toronto Press.

Rasmussen, H.M.D. and Rasmussen, B. (2012) 'Paradoxes in elder care: The Nordic model' in A. Kamp and H. Hvid (eds) *Elder care in Transition: Management, Meaning and Identity at Work: A Scandinavian Perspective*, Copenhagen: Copenhagen Business School Press, pp 29–50.

Region Sjælland (2016) *Vi er til for dig, Homepage*. [online] 22 November, Available from: www.regionsjaelland.dk [accessed 29 June 2021].

Smith, D.E. (2005) *Institutional Ethnography: A Sociology for People*, Lanham, New York, Toronto and Oxford: Altamira Press.

WHO (2016) *Patient Safety Assessment Mannual*, Regional Office for the Eastern Mediterranean, Cairo: WHO Library Cataloguing in Publication Data World. [online] 22 November, Available from: https://apps.who.int/iris/bitstream/handle/10665/249569/EMROPUB_2016_EN_18948.pdf?sequence=1&isAllowed=y [accessed 29 June 2021].

Wrede, S., Henriksson, L., Høst, H., Johansson, S. and Dybbroe, B. (eds) (2008) *Care Work in Crisis: Reclaiming the Nordic Ethos of Care*, Lund: Studentlitteratur.

8

Professionalisation of social pedagogues under managerial control: caring for children in a time of care crisis

Steen Baagøe Nielsen

Introduction

The field of early childhood education and care (ECEC) is characterised by great diversity in status and organisation in different countries. Care for children is commonly heavily dependent on unpaid and non-formal care work by mothers and relatives, or poorly paid nursing and child-minding, for instance by migrant workers (Acker, 1990; Bäck-Wiklund, 2004). Consequently, a common strategy for the valorisation of care work pursued by feminist policy-makers and researchers, in the Nordic countries in particular, is that of professionalisation or 'professional projects' (Witz, 1990; Williams, 1996; Dahl, 2010). In Denmark, this political strategy has been advocated not only by the labour unions of the (social, educational and health) care workers and by their educational institutions. The possibilities and advantages of professionalisation have also been taken up and promoted as part of policy discourses and regulatory reforms around the 'modernisation' of public services as a means to enhance the quality of care, and the legitimacy of public service and reproduction on a broader scale (Wrede et al, 2008; Dahl, 2010). Seen from this point of view, professionalisation is not a controversial strategy.

Taking a closer look at the underlying interests and explicit reasons for professionalisation, there is however less consensus among the advocating agents. In fact, discussions of professionalisation expose controversies not only about the *aims*, but also the *means* of professionalisation. Following Witz (1990), this chapter argues that the potential of professionalisation as a strategy rests on the validation of the substance of the professional practice at its core: on the one side, the basic understandings and recognition of the services rendered; on the other side, the status of professional knowledge, qualifications and necessary judgements, values and ethics needed to act with professionalism to secure the quality of the tasks and services provided. This chapter explores the potentials of professionalisation strategies, motivated by the central question of whether professionalisation will actually help in providing recognition for essential ECEC care work – and whether this can counteract a 'crisis of care', as discussed in the contributions to this book.

The following discussion will raise concerns about the status of care work and the potential of professionalisation based on empirical research in the context of care work in Danish ECECs. The term ECECs is used to denote the common public institutions in the field of ECEC. A central challenge for discussing the potential of greater recognition of care work through professionalisation strategies is the significance of contextual factors – here linked to the Danish/Nordic context and the public universal provision of ECECs as part of the Nordic welfare state model (Esping-Andersen, 1990). Much discussion of professions tends to be universal and/or functionalist, and therefore often becomes overshadowed by debates about the possibilities of professionalisation in light of general organisational dynamics and transformation of public services (that is, the administrative 'modernisation' influenced by New Public Management [NPM], for example Dahl, 2010). Though these insights are crucial, and will indeed inform the present discussion, the aim of this chapter is to highlight how the issue of professionalisation becomes highly complex and troublesome when seen in its specific institutional, political and practical context.

With a focus on Danish ECECs, the discussion considers the conditions and possibilities for recognition of care work. How do basic economic, social and organisational structures limit and shape both the possibilities of professionalisation of Danish 'social pedagogues' and the care work in childcare services in 'early years' (0–6 years)? The immediate focus is on the embedded obstacles and struggles, as well as the possibilities and barriers for professional recognition of this line of work.

To clarify the adopted theoretical and methodological position, on the current challenges of professionalisation, the chapter uses concepts that draw upon theories of professions, professionalism and professionalisation (Abbott, 1988; Witz, 1990; Evetts, 2003, 2009), but at the same time draws upon understandings of care work linked to the traditions of Nordic public service, and its modernisation (Wrede et al, 2008; Dahl, 2010). Crucially, this discussion takes place against the background of Fraser's focus on care crisis and boundary struggles (Fraser, 2013).

Professionalisation strategies and the care crisis

The fundamental conditions for the professionalisation of care are restricted and bounded not only by factors such as knowledge, judgement and ethics, but are also conditioned by the hierarchical position of reproductive work in relation to capitalist 'production', with care (as a commodity) positioned in a lower social and economic position. For Fraser, however, care work as social reproduction 'is an indispensable background condition for the possibility of economic production in a capitalist society' (Fraser, 2016: 102).

To grasp the particular Nordic context of the status and organisation of care work, the chapter supplements Fraser's understanding of care and 'care crisis' with theoretical understandings and insights from well-established fields of research and interesting theoretical and analytical perspectives of a tradition of Nordic care researchers (Wærness, 1984; Szebehely, 1995; Dahl et al, 2011).

Much of the research on care in the Anglo-American context has focused on the distinction between care (as 'women's work') and paid labour (where a 'male norm' is taken for granted). This is also partly the implied understanding of Fraser. Most Nordic research on care, however, has taken its starting point in the care work performed (mostly by women) within welfare institutions as waged labour. This research has extended the understanding of the complexities of the subordination of caring and care work, understood as 'social reproduction' in relation to 'production' in a capitalist society.

Central in Nordic care research are reflections around the consequences of a changing context of care work, developed within a feminist, multidisciplinary field of research. Most Nordic care researchers have thus explored the ways in which care and care work are both marginalised and made invisible as (social) production and undervalued as a source of wealth and well-being. The Nordic welfare states are characterised by broader gendered hierarchies and a lack of recognition tied to a universal and systemic 'gender order' (see Chapter 1 in this volume).

A central concern of Nordic care research has been to consider the possibilities and challenges of professionalising care work, as a way to transgress the subordinate position of care work. But complexities arise as the status of care work is linked to the regulation of the public sector(s), to changing care policies, as well as (particularly relevant for this chapter) the changing regimes of governance in the Nordic welfare states (Wærness, 1984; Szebehely, 1995; Baagøe Nielsen, 2006; Dahl, 2010, among others). Part of this research has been directly or indirectly related to ongoing attempts to professionalise care work. Care work is seen as a special kind of work; always already relational *and* personal. As a special kind of work – unlike the 'personal service' relations of consumerism – care work is understood to be organised as reciprocal relations involving the emotional engagement of the persons involved (Wærness, 1984; Martinsen, 2010). Likewise, the focus is on the ways in which the qualifications needed for such work extend beyond traditional educational credentials, by drawing upon a larger body of personal, emotional and empathic competencies, which are formed by informal experiences, socialisation and learning environments of personal relations, local communities and broader civil society. Further, Nordic care research has focused on the position of care work in a hierarchical cultural relation – considered as socially inferior and subordinate to men's 'proper', 'productive' work. Thus, the types of competencies needed are commonly understood to be inherently culturally gendered (Baagøe Nielsen and Westerling, 2014). As a result of such discourses, the qualities and 'results' of care work are made invisible, and the qualifications and knowledge it demands remain socially unrecognised or undervalued.

Through this well-established body of research on care work and the related theories of professionalism, this chapter explores particular challenges of care work professionalisation in the Nordic setting.

Perspectives on professionalisation

To understand the current challenges of professionalisation, this chapter draws on theories of professionalisation, in particular Evetts' distinction between organisational versus occupational professionalism (Evetts, 2009). This distinction seems particularly potent in a Nordic care context, as care work here is done mostly as waged labour by well-educated occupational or professional staff in public institutions, in stark contrast to traditions of privately organised, market-driven childcare (OECD, 2006, 2012).

To understand the status and legitimacy of professional services, most sociological theories of professions underline the importance of acquiring jurisdiction and the right or even monopoly to make autonomous judgement based on a foundation of academic knowledge. These in turn secure general recognition of a set of knowledge-based and specialised services based upon educational control and accepted social closure (for example Abbott, 1988; Witz, 1990; Eraut, 1994; Macdonald, 1995).

Seen from a traditional 'sociology of the professions' perspective it is, however, highly doubtful whether social pedagogues or any of the 'welfare professions' can be categorised as professions with their own jurisdiction and exclusive, knowledge-based social function. Therefore, other theories of professions are needed in order to understand the political attraction to the project of professionalisation, and its social and political trajectory. Evetts (2009) discusses the appeal and challenges embedded in the ideology of professionalism, separating between 'two different, contrasting ideal typical forms of professionalism' (Evetts, 2009: 248). Firstly, a traditional, *occupational professionalism* is built upon situational knowledge and collective and personal judgement. Trust is a central relational element, with authority being based on practitioner autonomy. Such authority, Evetts argues, 'depends on common and lengthy systems of education and vocational training and the development of strong occupational identities and work cultures' (Evetts, 2009: 248). Crucially, controls are operationalised by practitioners themselves. Evetts contrasts this with *organisational professionalism* that is manifested by a discourse of control that incorporates rational–legal forms of authority and hierarchical structures of responsibility and decision-making. Other characteristics are increasingly standardised work procedures, external managerial forms of regulation and accountability measures, for example target-setting and performance review (Evetts, 2009: 248). Though elements of this strategy seem to employ an ideology of professionalism at its core it neglects the experience and workplace-based knowledge that practitioners carry and control themselves. It denies them their right to use this knowledge and their collective, occupational knowledge to make personal, situational judgement.

The status of care work with children in the Nordic countries: professionalisation under siege?

International organisations such as UNESCO and the OECD in particular (OECD, 2006, 2012) have over the last decades argued for stronger institutional foundations and the need for qualified staff not only in pre-school services, but also in less formalised ECECs, such as for very young children in crèches (0–2 year olds).

In the Nordic countries, the universal provision of publicly organised and financed services has changed the field of childcare into a more professionalised field of work. This means that a small majority of the care workers are today 'social pedagogues' with bachelor degrees as formal qualifications. The field also employs around 35 to 45 per cent of assistant pedagogues, either without or with few formal qualifications, including a larger number of home-based child-minders.

The ideals of autonomous and highly valorised professional services have formed the underlying and sometimes explicit goals of several Danish unions of 'welfare workers' to formulate professionalisation strategies through the 1990s and 2000s especially, in a period of intensified political and administrative (bureaucratic) rationalisation of care work, as well as intensified educational reform. In Denmark, the nurses' union was a frontrunner for this in 1992, the teachers' union followed in 2002 and the social workers' union in 2006. The Danish National Federation of Early Childhood Teachers and Youth Educators (BUPL) formulated and approved their first strategy for professionalisation in 2004.

Social care work has not only been a field of professionalisation but also of 'boundary struggles' around the status and recognition of childcare and education as such (Fraser, 2013). Central actors, such as the unions, argue that a project of professionalisation will secure a genuinely knowledge-based practice, higher recognition, better working conditions, better salaries and as a consequence higher quality of care (BUPL, 2006).

The formulation of these professionalisation strategies coincided between 2000 and 2010 with extensive educational reforms, which turned the foundational education for most of the care and reproductive work into bachelor degree programmes, linked to the merger of more than 200 educational institutions into only six 'professional colleges'. These colleges have become strong political agents, promoting professionalism through academisation. This institutional reframing of educational programmes has been decisive in a discursive change in which the practitioners began to understand themselves as professionals (Jensen, 2004; Baagøe Nielsen and Bøje, 2018). In the years to follow it became commonplace, if not obligatory, to identify central welfare service jobs such as teachers, nurses, social workers and social pedagogues as professionals. For most of the involved institutional actors both within these huge sectors of 'welfare service work' and within the new powerful educational institutions qualifying new social pedagogues, this was considered an 'upgrading'. Following international trends and the Bologna Process, they campaigned for proper academic status and lobbied for state-granted research funds hitherto reserved for the universities to make their programmes research based (Baagøe Nielsen and Bøje, 2018).

At the same time, this push towards professionalisation was seen as a way to create a certain distance from earlier notions and discourses of bureaucratic arrogance and self-interest (du Gay, 2000), while on the other hand establishing a distance from discourses of a 'calling' as basic motivation for care work. The aim was to push for more academically qualified knowledge-based education. The new discursive framing of these 'street-level bureaucrats' or 'frontline workers' was neither seen as controversial nor problematic from a state and public employer perspective. Quite on the contrary, it was actively promoted though the employers had been less precise of other aims of professionalisation than expectations of more 'value for money'.

To understand why the new framing of welfare workers as professionals was accepted and even promoted by the state, this needs to be considered as a strategy within the overall political-administrative reforms often named 'modernisation' (Baagøe Nielsen, 2006; Kamp and Hvid, 2012).

The 'modernisation' discourse would itself promote a specific type of professionalisation through its major focus on the 'right to choose' between different services in the pursuit of 'value for money'. The idea was to enable clients, users and 'citizens, 'released' from former one-string, 'monopolised' service provision, to choose the services they prefer on a free market, thus rendering it legitimate to close down services not in demand. Public management and the political-administrative level have over the past decades acted more and more as employers in the market. Therefore, they should hardly be expected to support the 'professional project' of setting up new strategies of exclusionary qualification, ethical standards, authorisation and/

or monopolisation of central functions, which would convey a rise of social status and qualitative standards adding to the 'knowledge mandate' as political mobilisation and influence (Witz, 1990). On the contrary these transformations in the institutional set-up and in the field of practice in Danish ECECs seem only to enable strategies of *organisational professionalisation* (Evetts, 2009) rather than that of a traditional *occupational* 'professional project' (Witz, 1990). As Witz (1990) have previously pointed out, such 'female professional projects' are further challenged as they are ultimately dependant on the recognition within traditional patriarchal structures.

Organisational and managerial reform in the ECECs

In Denmark, the ECEC-field has been marked by many other developments than those directly linked to professionalisation (Dahl et al, 2011). There have been changes in the local organisation of ECECs, with merging of institutions to larger units and a strengthening of the positions of local managers, who are encouraged to take generic management courses tailored to a range of different institutions, despite the fact that the allegiances of the local ECEC managers, who are all social pedagogues themselves, have traditionally been with the staff rather than the administrative bodies. Further, there has been widespread establishment of policies that invite international contractors to sell their programmes, concepts and procedures to be implemented and applied in public institutions. Many of these initiatives have been followed by hitherto unwanted accountability measures for practice (Aabro, 2016). In the political and managerial bodies of public administration, this agenda is not seen as being at odds with an agenda of professionalisation, but rather as two sides of a coin which will both add to the 'quality' of the services. Evetts warns that the focus on output measures and productivity, as part of organisational professionalisation, might turn a blind eye to more traditional and well-established understandings of quality in work practices: 'The work organization's managerial demands for quality control and audit, for target setting and performance review become reinterpreted as promoting professionalism itself' (Evetts, 2009: 254).

The Danish social pedagogic tradition and its challenges

It is a particular characteristic of the Nordic countries that this framing of social reproduction, and the disregard and silencing of those performing the tasks it entails, has especially since the 1960s been challenged and supplemented by a massive transformation of care work to be part of universal 'public services'. Childcare services are provided by the state as a universal right, paid and organised by municipalities, managing and supporting the local institutions (Borchorst, 2000; Eydal and Rostgaard, 2010).

At the same time, Danish ECECs have long been acknowledged for maintaining a fruitful 'social pedagogic tradition' in the EU, UNESCO and OECD. This rather holistic tradition, shared with a number of other Nordic countries and parts of Germany, has been acknowledged as an alternative to an 'early education' or 'pre-primary' approach primarily concerned with formal curricular activities and expectations of explicit learning outcomes as direct preparation for school. Influential OECD reviews (OECD, 2006, 2012) praised especially the Danish services as they seemed to provide for dual-earner families, higher birth-rates, and a good learning space for children (see also Bäck-Wiklund, 2004; Baagøe Nielsen, 2014).

Likewise, Denmark's ECECs have received recognition for their high quality, understood as a low ratio of children per staff member, well-educated professional staff, affordable provision, reasonable learning outcomes, high parental involvement, and so on. The OECD especially stressed the qualities of the social pedagogic, 'holistic' tradition to be about the care and upbringing, as well as learning, of young children – rather than an early childhood specialist or a (pre-school) teacher tied to a fixed 'curriculum' (OECD, 2006: 163ff). The social pedagogue is trained to take a wider view of early learning and the importance of free play, and is trained to understand the role of ECEC in the wider field of society. The OECD highlights and supports the caring and 'holistic' orientation, with a focus on 'supporting children in their current developmental tasks and interests' (OECD, 2006: 57), but seems to downplay that this tradition is linked to explicit encouragement of children's 'free play' and their active participation and involvement as democratic citizens.

The severe and complex qualitative implication for the children of the current transformations are not the issue for this chapter, but it is apparent that while some researchers are concerned (for example Gitz-Johansen, 2019), such institutional 'alignments' are commonly acknowledged as necessary in the light of a more general cultural and social transformation of the social reproduction of modern societies. The reforms are linked not only to a call for rationalisation but also to the rise of a more genuine common political interest in childhood as a necessary social investment (Heckman, 2006), resulting in an intensified political and organisational interest in the work of the social pedagogues as they are partly at odds with the holistic traditions. The care work in ECEC institutions are now increasingly discursively framed as a 'learning pedagogy'; sometimes playful but most often with a focus on didactic organisation to stimulate the cognitive competences of the child (Baagøe Nielsen, 2014).

While this pedagogic orientation towards cognitive stimulation has always been a part of the Nordic tradition in childcare and 'social pedagogy' (Vejleskov, 1997; Baagøe Nielsen, 2006, 2014), there is no doubt that the emphasis has grown significantly over the last ten years. The introduction of state-imposed and regulated curricula to be enforced and implemented through a chain of command, through local municipalities and institutional managers, has transformed the care work of the social pedagogues at the individual institution. Some argue that this has threatened the fundamental values of social pedagogy and resulted in increasingly formal and instrumental, rather than empathetic and child-centred, relations, further reducing the quality of the pedagogues' practice and limiting the importance of their traditional knowledge base (Ahrenkiel et al, 2013; Togsverd, 2015).

Knowledge produced far from care practices or the relevant ECEC institution, notably in international monitoring bodies such as the OECD, intervenes and affects the social status and legitimacy of the practices of social pedagogues. This legitimises a change of focus from core practices and local knowledge and establishes care work as waged labour at the lower end of the pay scale and common social-status hierarchy. It allows for different types of institutionalised forms of disrespect (Dahl, 2010). At the same time, a course of professionalisation is not denied at the managerial level, but simply understood to mean more rational organisation, providing a better quality of services. This is not achieved by strengthening the autonomy, recognition and status of the judgements of the professions, but by managerial organisation of more rational or 'lean' practices; if not by simply removing the qualitative elements of traditional social pedagogical judgement, much along the lines of Evetts' (2009) organisational professionalisation.

The political pressures and new managerial and formal framing of this type of institution result in extensive changes to this specific type of care work, which challenges basic understandings of social pedagogy to the core, causing a double-sided challenge to the social pedagogues' union when pursuing a strategy of professionalisation.

Early childhood education and care as care work in crisis

The complex qualities of the work of social pedagogues in ECECs cannot be measured in terms of 'productivity' or 'learning outcomes', that is, the ability to produce learning for children according to some (perhaps even progressive) curriculum. Instead, it is essential to also look into the ways in which ECEC provides for social justice and equality on a broader scale. Following Fraser's framework, read through a Nordic care research perspective, social pedagogues are based within a capitalist mode of production, which fundamentally challenges, and is at odds with, the actual needs of the carer as well as the children. This crisis of care continuously affects and threatens the status of care work. It systematically distorts our understanding of the tasks involved in care work and reduces the understanding of the body of knowledge needed for care workers to engage in necessary work. In linking the discussion about professionalisation and the care crisis, this section outlines the importance of focusing on the resulting inequalities, that is, the inequality of status, priority, and control of the working conditions.

Much of the problems that arise around the attempted professionalisation of care work can still be explained within the theoretical framework that labels this care work as semi-professional with limited possibilities of acquiring real jurisdiction and autonomy through an 'occupational closure' within a patriarchal, capitalist society (Witz, 1990). Care work in ECEC is still also gendered, reflecting broader gendered patterns of the care crisis. Only around 7 per cent of the educated social pedagogues are male, and though men often constitute up to 25 per cent of the assistant staff, there is still a very common understanding of the gender(ing) of this type of work, which challenges the recruitment of men, and reminds (other) men that this is not proper and well-paid work (Baagøe Nielsen, 2011).

In Denmark as well as in the other Nordic countries, much of the care work for children has been transformed into paid labour in the public sector. Well above 80 per cent of all women aged between 25 and 40 are working, and the labour activity rates are thus almost on a par with those of men a few percentage points higher. This means that more than 95 per cent of children from the age of 10–12 months up to the age of 5 will spend on average 7.5 hours, five days a week in an ECEC facility. Public day-care facilities can almost be seen as obligatory as most family need dual careers, not only to satisfy their personal ambitions but also as a matter of maintaining basic living conditions. In most parts of the country, you cannot as parents pay for even a modest house without a dual income, and if you should feel that your child needs you more, you will experience that the almost universal reality of the dual-earner family leaves streets and playgrounds empty with no one to play with.

Despite the general sympathy in the OECD to the 'holistic tradition' mentioned earlier, the NPM-led governing agendas included in the OECD reports nevertheless ask for the implementation of more exact performance indicators (OECD, 2006). Their recommendations (in 2006 and 2007) entail an explicit and powerful quest for quality as 'performance to be measured' – and they highlight the need to improve policies and establish 'good practice' through the implementation of the NPM tools.

Thus, the OECD has, over the last ten years, encouraged a shift of focus towards the use of more audit and assessment, through the provision of tools for monitoring and increasing the quality in ECEC. These tools include key performance indicators, output controls, and monitoring linked to accountability measure goals, allowing benchmarking of further competition among services. Such external evaluation and control measures are ultimately based on an instrumentalist approach far from the holistic, occupational traditions of ECECs. The new regime establishes control and disciplining mechanisms beyond the autonomous judgement and practices of care workers. It breaks the traditional bond of high trust, and the autonomy to

Table 8.1: Change of working conditions in ECECs: child–staff ratios

	1986	2000	2010	2014
Child–adult ratio (0–2 years)	4,1	5,2	6,2	6,5
Child–adult ratio (3–6 years)	7,5	9,7	11,4	11,8
Share of hours (%) used with children	67%	56.7%	51%	51%

Source: Bureau2000 (2018)

make local, holistic judgements building on respect in the collegial relations, and cooperation with and support from the children's parents.

Partly as a result of these regulatory trends, the working conditions which should provide for this type of care in ECECs have deteriorated. This is made obvious by the direct cuts in the means allocated per child, but also, notably, by the growing number of hours spent on 'other activities' than contact with the children such as monitoring and assessment, as well as other types of bureaucracy and managerial tasks.

Table 8.1 provides an overview of the increase in the child-staff ratio in ECECs in Denmark from 1986 to 2014. Considering that the hours spent directly with the children has decreased, these figures point to a real decrease of hours spent on pedagogical activities with the child of almost 30 per cent since 2000, and almost 80 per cent since 1986. There is much public debate that this ratio has now become dangerously low, manifesting, for example, in the 'Hvor er der en voksen?' campaign ('Where can I find an adult?'). Since the 2019 election and a new left majority, the priorities of this field finally seem to be increasing slightly again.

Care in Danish ECECs under pressure: voices from the floor and classroom

This situation has created intensified pressure on staff. A research project, which focused on the competencies of the newly graduated pedagogues, found an overwhelming sense of frustration and even disillusionment among most of them (Baagøe Nielsen and Bøje, 2018). Helene's voice here is exemplary of our general findings:

'I didn't know much about day care facilities, so I just had to jump right into it, and I have to admit … that during the first few months, I thought: "I simply cannot manage this!"

And I know very well that in the crèche [where most of her colleagues work] staff ratios are different … but here in the kindergarten [3–6 years] we are often alone in the peripheral hours [early morning and late afternoon], with up to 22 children in a [class]room.

Being on your own, you can consider and try out whether you can "deliver" anything educational at all: and you can't! You just cannot manage, right!?'

Newly graduated staff express feelings of helplessness, frustration and even of shock as a result of their transition from education to being a social pedagogue in the workplace. Whereas the so-called 'practice shock' or transition shock is widely described among nurses and teachers (Kramer, 1974; Veenman, 1984; Eraut, 1994), it has not previously been observed among social pedagogues in Denmark. The problem as described by the newly graduated pedagogues is not only one of stress and heavy pressures put upon them by the continuing worsening of working conditions, combined with the rising demands of professionalisation. It is exacerbated by the difficulties of finding full-time employment as a social pedagogue; many of the positions available have been reduced to 25 or 30 hours per week due to economic 'rationalisations'. Another central strain on Helene's care work was the fact that the legitimacy of holistic pedagogy seemed to have dwindled. Therefore, Helene was, as with others of the other newly graduated pedagogues we observed and interviewed, particularly anxious to promote and do 'educational work according to plan'. In order to do this, Helene attempted to take time out, around 20 to 30 minutes per day, away from the children, to prepare a 'toolbox programme', an evidence-based anti-bullying programme. Despite her normal workday of six to seven hours, she saw this curricular activity as her main legitimising activity. Helene found this very helpful, especially in securing the support of the parents, who found this introduction of a strictly curriculum-based programme meaningful.

Central to the holistic pedagogical approach is the importance of working organically, in the German tradition, 'vom Kinde aus', that is, with a starting point in the motivation and activities of the individual child, to address the collective interests and ideas of the children as a group, and thus, also from a democratic intention perspective, to facilitate real involvement and genuine influence of the children (Brembeck et al, 2004). This understanding demands local autonomy for the practitioner, in order to be able to make contextually based judgements. The legitimacy of such a practice rests both on a fluid and situational pedagogy, and a contextual understanding of good practice, rather than a strict, pre-set curriculum. This has been described as a 'pedagogy of everyday practices' with a strong focus on the pedagogical element of care practices. More often than not, these are (formally) unnoticed (Ahrenkiel et al, 2013) or, as feminist care research argues, even deliberately marginalised and 'made invisible' (Szebehely, 1995; Baagøe Nielsen, 2006). The competencies needed for this type of holistic social pedagogy require not only the right and authority to make autonomous situational judgements, but also depend on individual and collective development of strong occupational identities and work cultures, which rest not only on a lengthy system of vocational education and training, but must be maintained through a legitimate reflexive practice among colleagues, who are involved in operationalising the necessary improvements and developments of these practice themselves.

An excerpt from our observation protocol registering Helene's professional practice in a day-care facility room showed the following typical episode:

This morning Helene's hours are used, for example, to bring the children toys from the shelves that they cannot reach themselves; talk to Karen (support pedagogue) about a specific child, who has problems; discipline the children if they get too loud, or they have conflicts, tease one another, etc.

In between, she must attend to other needs – if, for example, a child has a cough, and Helene will need to call the parents to come and pick up the child; another child will come and sit on her lap, and Helene will nuzzle her hair and say 'my darling'.

Further, she will need to spend time cleaning up – and making the children clean up. Cleaning up goes on continuously, so that the tiny [class]room can be used for many functions. However, cleaning up is particularly necessary when lunchtime approaches. Now, Helene speaks in a highly authoritative voice to make the children clean up and get ready for lunch.

This excerpt indicates a common practice in an ECEC, which entails a number of pedagogical possibilities, but also, on this busy day, contains the need for authoritative, situational judgement. As a newly graduated social pedagogue, Helene finds this type of practice not only stressful but almost without genuine pedagogical value, though this type of practice is much more common than the pre-structured pedagogical activities. We see the emergence of a new pedagogical division between the formal, which is monitored and valued, such as learning activities, and broader measurable tasks on the one hand, and the majority of 'unnoticed' everyday activities on the other. Over the last decades, the field has witnessed a formalisation which tends to render many of the necessary daily, trivial tasks even more 'invisible': the provision for physical needs, cleaning up, comforting or directing a child and so on – the kind of work that never stops, and which you can hardly measure.

The standpoint of the defenders of the holistic tradition is that caring for children, providing for their well-being and learning can never solely and durably be understood (or measured) by monitoring learning outcomes. Instead, to succeed in caring relations all the involved parties, parents, professionals and children, must be heard, understood and acknowledged as necessary contributors. A focus on monitoring children's learning, rather than their well-being or the quality of their care relations, removes important ethical, relational and democratic aspects of the work. Work-life research within care work points to the fact that formalisation and lack of relational responsiveness tends to silence real care needs, with an accompanying tendency to routinise and standardise the work-life of carers (Baagøe Nielsen, 2011).

The professionalisation of social pedagogues: a double-edged sword

As discussed in this chapter, a central understanding of governance practice in NPM is that of creating controllable effects through standardisation and 'best practice'. This idea often depends on the implementation of standards and technologies of knowledge built on the understanding of evidence-based practice. Though this might be effective in the short run, the standardisation of procedures cannot replace workplace-based, relational knowledge and the necessary situational judgements by well-educated professionals. The results of 'evidence-based' programmes, and the many extra monitoring practices they imply, are not convincing on their own terms. And, as highlighted, they do take up time which could be spent with the children.

Monitoring of services is implicitly (or sometimes explicitly) supported in order to support marketisation of services, as it becomes easier to make open tenders in (so-called) open competition when the services are closely described and allow for detailed monitoring. Simple indicators on output measures make it possible for commercial bidders and contractors to post and brand their results in competition with publicly financed institutions. Even in the Nordic countries, we see an increased commercialisation of care and education for children (see also Chapter 1 in this volume). This will often further an erosion of the privileges of public financing, lead to further segregation of the workforce and increasing managerialism within the institution, and turn care work into affective work, simply for commercial gain (Shirin Rai and Thomas, 2013).

Hopes have been high in Denmark (as in many other countries) that any type of professionalisation and public commitment to the provision of quality childcare and education would bring more attention to the field, and further recognition of the knowledge-based work there. It has been argued that further pressure for closer monitoring practices or more vivid engagement in local evaluations will make the already existing firmly knowledge-based practice 'visible' and noticed (Danmarks Evalueringsinstitut, 2017); this would then bring about a new respect and status for the care workers (BUPL, 2006). If 'professionalisation', however, means adapting already established evidence-based practice, and 'transparent competence' means simply complying with pre-organisational evidence-based standards and procedures, this will undoubtedly *diminish* the autonomy of the professionals. Working conditions will accordingly be experienced as poorer, which is in fact a path of *de*professionalisation and *de*skilling of work, rather than one of upgrading. In this way, professionalisation through *organisational professionalisation* strategies might be seen as another way of silencing the interest of carers, of women – and of traditional caring knowledge.

In a recent generational study on changes in the knowledge and practices of social pedagogues (Krøjer et al, 2017), the younger generation of social pedagogues in particular made quite clear the administrative and monitoring pressures they feel in their daily work, which affect their self-esteem and status with the parents:

Eva: I feel a certain sadness to have to spent so much time and effort to give them what they want [the administration or sometimes the parents]. To put the right marks on the right activities – as we are asked to do. And then there is only the remaining hours to be with the children.

Jacob: If you don't understand that you need to comply, you are considered 'not really flexible and innovative'. They [the bureaucrats] might be tolerant at first but after a while they will make you understand!

Lia: The parents will attempt to set high standards, and demand us to comply with latest scientific results they have come across … I will often disagree in silence: 'Have they ever witnessed the daily lives of kids in a child care facility?' But I try to use their [the parent's] show of interest for the best.

The consequence of pursuing the path of professionalisation might very well entail social pedagogues' necessary adjustments to a more standardised practice – followed by what might be termed 'a double discourse' around their jobs and tasks in which they will 'officially' have to stand up for the slogans of professionalism, but in fact must find their own ways to pursue real quality of practice.

Conclusion

This chapter has argued for broader recognition of the qualities in the work of childcare, through other paths than formalisation and organisational professionalisation. The double-edged sword of the 'professionalisation discourse' leads to further undermining of care work, which has historically been based on women's labour and competencies within a strong pedagogic tradition (Baagøe Nielsen, 2006). One tendency here seems to be that a minor portion of the 'professionals' will be drawn into managerial positions to legitimate the demands of parents and policy-makers, while the professionalisation discourse will serve to transform most of the work into routinised labour.

So far, the parents of children enrolled have been advocates and allies for a continuous focus on the quality of relational and situational care. The growing focus on the well-being of pre-school children has gained further traction over the last years and has thus added to the general public and political interest in the field. Perhaps the trends within the families towards generative fathering, and the engagement of men in the daily care, could be a new starting point for this discussion (Baagøe Nielsen and Westerling, 2014). This might not only benefit the women who (still most often) do the care work, it will most likely also enhance the conditions for the children (and their families) in need of care.

On a more methodological level, this chapter has highlighted the need for a contextual awareness of the limited gains following a strategy of organisational 'professionalisation'. A key argument laid out in the chapter is for a strengthened focus on the actual practical conditions of care work (that is, its formalisation, academisation and instrumentalisation), and the need for a continued focus on the persistent but also transformative structural conditions of caring and reproduction, and the new challenge this presents. These challenges, the chapter argues, may partly be explored through materialist feminist inquiry, but – following also the Nordic care research – these insights need to be complemented by more contextual and 'cultural' understandings of the dynamics of professionalisation to fully grasp the complex reproduction of patriarchal reductions of the value of care work.

References

Aabro, C. (2016) *Koncepter i pædagogisk arbejde*, Copenhagen: Hans Reitzels Forlag.

Abbott, A. (1988) *The System of the Professions*, London: University of Chicago Press.

Acker, J. (1990) 'Hierarchies, jobs and bodies: A theory of gendered organizations', *Gender & Society*, 4(1): 39–58.

Ahrenkiel, A., Baagøe Nielsen, S., Schmidt, C., Sommer, F. and Warring, N. (2013) *Daginstitutionsarbejde og pædagogisk faglighed*, Frederiksberg: Frydenlund.

Baagøe Nielsen, S. (2006) *Mænd og daginstitutionsarbejdets modernisering— Teoretiske, historiske og etnografiske perspektiver på sammenhænge mellem køn, pædagogisk arbejde og organisering i daginstitutioner*, Roskilde: Roskilde University.

Baagøe Nielsen, S. (ed) (2011) *Nordiske mænd til omsorgsarbejde! En forskningsbaseret erfaringsopsamling på initiativer til at rekruttere, uddanne og fastholde mænd efter finanskrisen*, Roskilde: Roskilde University.

Baagøe Nielsen, S. (2014) 'Daginstitutionernes skiftende politiske mandat' in J. Krejsler, A. Ahrenkiel and C. Schmidt (eds) *Kampen om daginstitutionen*, Frederiksberg: Frydenlund Academic, pp 71–95.

Baagøe Nielsen, S. and Bøje, J. (eds) (2018) *Attraktiv på papiret? Nyuddannede pædagoger mellem akademisering, vidensbasering professionalisering og omsorgsfuld praksisudvikling*, Velpro. Center for Velfærd, Profession og Hverdagsliv, Roskilde: Roskilde universitetscenter.

Baagøe Nielsen, S. and Westerling, A. (2014) 'Fathering as a learning process: Breaking new grounds in familiar territory' in G.B. Eydal and T. Rostgaard (eds) *Fatherhood in the Nordic Welfare States: Comparing Care Policies and Practice*, Bristol: Policy Press, pp 187–208.

Bäck-Wiklund, M. (2004) 'Nye tendenser i tidsfælden – Sverige som case' in M.II. Jacobsen and J. Tonboe (eds) *Arbejdssamfundet*, Copenhagen: Hans Reitzels Forlag, pp 131–151.

Borchorst, A. (2000) 'Den danske børnepasningsmodel – kontinuitet og forandring', *Arbejderhistorie*, 4: 55–69.

Brembeck, H., Johansson, B. and Kampmann, J. (eds) (2004) *Beyond the Competent Child: Exploring Contemporary Childhoods in the Nordic Welfare Societies*, Frederiksberg: Samfundslitteratur.

BUPL (2006) *The Work of the Pedagogue: Roles and Tasks*, Available from: https://bupl.dk/wp-content/uploads/2018/02/publikationer-the_work_of_the_pedagogue.pdf [accessed 10 September 2020].

Bureau 2000 (2018) *Børn pr. voksen i daginstitutioner – udviklingen 1972–2018*, Available from: www.bureau2000.dk/CustomerData/Files/Folders/7-seneste-nyheder/1081_b%C3%B8rn-pr-voksen-0511-2019.pdf [accessed 10 September 2020].

Dahl, H.M. (2010) 'An old map of state feminism and an insufficient recognition of care', *NORA – Nordic Journal of Feminist and Gender Research*, 18(3): 152–166.

Dahl, H.M., Keränen, M. and Kovalainen, A. (2011) 'Introduction' in H.M. Dahl, M. Keränen and A. Kovalainen (eds) *Europeanization, Care and Gender: Global Complexities*, London: Palgrave Macmillan, pp 13–29.

Danmark Evalueringsinstitut (2017) Udvikling i ledelse på dagtilbudsområdet. Notat. Available from: https://www.eva.dk/dagtilbud-boern/udvikling-ledelse-paa-dagtibudsomraadet [accessed 10 September 2020].

du Gay, P. (2000) *In Praise of Bureaucracy: Weber, Organisation, Ethics*, London: Sage.

Eraut, M. (1994) *Developing Professional Knowledge and Competence*, London: RoutledgeFalmer.

Eriksen, T.R. (2004) 'Gendered professional identity and professional knowledge in female health education: Put into perspective by a follow-up study (1987–2002)', *NORA*, 12(1): 20–30.

Esping-Andersen, G. (1990) *The Three Worlds of Welfare Capitalism*, Cambridge: Polity Press.

Evetts, J. (2003) 'The sociological analysis of professionalism: Occupational change in the modern world', *International Sociology*, 18(2): 395–415.

Evetts, J. (2009) 'A new professionalism? Challenges and opportunities', *Current Sociology*, 59(4): 406–422.

Eydal, G.B. and Rostgaard, T. (2010) 'På vej mod en nordisk børnepasnings-politik – hvad var de politiske processer og dagsordner?' in I.V. Gislason (ed) *Foräldraledighet, omsorgspolitik och jamställdhet i Norden*, København: Nordisk Ministerråd, pp 135–169.

Fraser, N. (2013) *Fortunes of Feminism: From State-Managed Capitalism to Neoliberal Crisis*, London and New York: Verso.

Fraser, N. (2016) 'Contradictions of capital and care', *New Left Review*, 100: 99–117.

Gitz-Johansen, T.G. (2019) *Vuggestueliv – Omsorg, følelser og relationer*, Frederiksberg: Samfundslitteratur.

Heckman, J. (2006) 'Skill formation and the economics of investing in disadvantaged children', *Science*, 312(5782): 1900–1902.

Jensen, K. (ed) (2004) *Professionsfagenes krise – en udfordring til lærer-, pædagog- og sygeplejeskeuddannelserne*, Copenhagen: Danmarks Pædagogiske Universitets Forlag.

Kamp, A. and Hvid, H. (ed) (2012) *Elder care in transition: Management, meaning and identity at work. A Scandinavian perspective*, Copenhagen: Business School Press.

Kramer, M. (1974) *Reality Shock: Why Nurses Leave Nursing*, St. Louis: C.V. Mosby.

Krøjer, J., Baagøe Nielsen, S. and Mogensen, K.H. (2017) 'Generationsspecifikke forskelle mellem pædagogers faglighed', *Tidsskrift for Arbejdsliv*, 19(4): 74–88.

Macdonald, K.H. (1995) *The Sociology of the Professions*, London: SAGE.

Martinsen, K. (2010) *Øjet og Kaldet* (2nd edn), København: Munksgaard.

OECD (2006) *Starting Strong II: Early Childhood Education and Care*, Paris: OECD Publishing, Available from: www.oecd.org/education/school/startingstrongiiearlychildhoodeducationandcare.htm [accessed 10 September 2020].

OECD (2012) *Starting Strong III: A Quality Toolbox for Early Childhood Education and Care*, Paris: OECD Publishing.

Shirin Rai, C.H. and Thomas, D. (2013) 'Depletion: The cost of social reproduction', *International Feminist Journal of Politics*, 16(1): 86–105.

Szebehely, M. (1995) *Vardagens organisering: om vårdbiträden och gamla i hemtjänsten*, Lund Studies in Social Welfare IX, Lund: Arkiv förlag.

Togsverd, L. (2015) *Da kvaliteten kom til småbørnsinstitutionerne*, PhD thesis, Roskilde: Roskilde University.

Veenman, S.A.M. (1984) 'Perceived problems of beginning teachers', *Review of Educational Research*, 54(2): 143–178.

Vejleskov, H. (ed) (1997) *Den danske børnehave – studier om myter, meninger og muligheder*, Skrifter fra Center for Småbørnsforskning no. 8, Vejle: Kroghs Forlag.

Wærness, K. (1984) 'The rationality of caring', *Economic and Industrial Democracy*, 5(2): 185–211.

Williams, C. (1996) *Still a Man's World: Men Who Do 'Women's Work'*, Los Angeles: University of California Press.

Witz, A. (1990) 'Patriarchy and professions: The gendered politics of occupational closure', *Sociology*, 24(4): 675–690.

Wrede, S., Henriksson, L., Høst, H., Johansson, S. and Dybbroe, B. (eds) (2008) 'Introduction: Care work and the competing rationalities of public policy' in S. Wrede, L. Henriksson, H. Høst, S. Johansson and B. Dybbroe (eds) *Care Work in Crisis: Reclaiming the Nordic Ethos of Care*, Lund: Studentlitteratur, pp 15–37.

9

Raising quality in Norwegian early childhood centres: (re)producing the care crisis?

Birgitte Ljunggren

Introduction

The care crisis arises from the contradictions between the capitalist society's dependence on social reproduction (caring) and mechanisms in capitalist organisations that undermine the very reproduction on which they depend (Fraser, 2016). Work organisations can in their quest for profit, legitimacy or efficiency, be organised in ways that hamper the combination of childcare and paid work for parents, or self-care for employees. This happens despite the fact that organisations themselves rely on well-functioning labour power premised by social reproduction. Acker (2006) describes the one-sided organisational focus on supporting and enhancing production as a corporate non-responsibility towards caring. The high degree of early childhood education and care (ECEC) coverage and public financing of Nordic ECEC services (Karila, 2012) implies that early childhood centres, organisations, play a vital role in social reproduction. Currently, 91.3 per cent of all Norwegian children aged 1–5 attend early childhood centres (ECCs) (Statistics Norway, 2020a). This chapter explores traces of the care crisis in Norwegian ECCs, approaching them as work organisations set to produce high-quality care by raising staff competence in cost-efficient ways.

Publicly financed full-time ECEC lies at the heart of the care crisis not only because it transfers care work from parents to organisations, and thereby allows parents the combination of paid work and care. ECCs shall produce high-quality care and education that is regarded as the foundation for citizens' future labour market participation and national economic growth (Segerholm, 2012). This quality turn is also evident in Norwegian ECEC policy (Ljunggren and Lauritzen, 2018). Lacking competence as a source for low quality is highlighted by OECD reports on the Norwegian ECEC sector (Engel et al, 2015) and is further repeated in the current national strategy for competence raising and recruitment (Ministry of Education and Research, 2017b). This strategy strongly supports a model for raising competence within the ECCs that includes staff in common reflections, co-creation and collaboration with external knowledge suppliers. Subsequently, leaders and staff shall use their work time on guidance and to co-construct learning.

The quality of Norwegian ECCs remains in question, and others have pointed at a lack of organisational capacity as a source of low ECEC quality (Ljunggren et al, 2017). Capacity refers to available time and time-use in ECCs and are organisational factors. Norwegian case studies have documented workdays marked by high intensity, demand for efficiency and little slack (Enehaug et al, 2008; Nicolaisen et al, 2012). In Danish ECCs Monrad (2017) finds that care work takes form of self-governance that individualises work responsibilities in times of cutbacks. This indicates that ECCs are *meagre organisations*, who have a scarcity of resources compared to their assigned tasks (Trägårdh and Lindberg, 2004). In sum this suggests that the care crisis is reproduced in ECCs, and its features will be further explored in this chapter. The current chapter answers the need for research on care as it is understood within organisational frames. Aslanian (2017) calls for a broader understanding of care in ECEC that relates to organisational aspects. There is scarce research on the relationship between competence-raising schemes and the care crisis in Norwegian ECCs. Such competence-raising processes are potential time thieves since they might add new tasks that are not necessarily supported by sufficient capacity. This might represent a social reproductive contradiction (Fraser, 2016) in Norwegian ECCs that I explore with the following research questions:

- Do we find traces of the care crisis in Norwegian ECCs in the wake of introducing competence raising as a quality measure?
- How do ECC leaders and employees answer the care crisis, and what are the preconditions for those answers?

To elaborate these questions I apply organisational theory about time, to analyse data from two datasets on ECC-based competence schemes. Such theory is suitable to operationalise the social-reproductive contradiction of capitalism.

Background: Norwegian early childhood centres

All Norwegian ECCs are legally required to follow the Kindergarten Act and the Framework Plan (Ministry of Education and Research, 2017a). These regulations reflect the Norwegian ECEC as being part of a Nordic ECEC tradition that integrates care, play and learning in ECEC practices (Karila, 2012). Care intertwines with pedagogical practices in ECEC; however, I attempt to maintain a particular focus on caring since it is a premise for child well-being, learning and development in this tradition (Eidevald and

Engdahl, 2018). Even though the Norwegian ECEC field is marked by institutionalised diversity in ownership, this does not seem to affect the content of the service in large degree (Haugset, 2018).

Staff structure in Norwegian ECCs consists of directors, pedagogical leaders, skilled assistants (who have a certificate of apprenticeship) and unskilled assistants. Directors and pedagogical leaders are required to have a formal education with at least a bachelor level degree that qualifies them for pedagogical work with children. Directors ensure that the pedagogical work complies with the Framework Plan, and the pedagogical leaders are responsible for the didactical work and guiding the skilled and unskilled assistants' work with the children. They have the responsibility to turn ECCs into learning organisations (Ministry of Education and Research, 2011).

According to Statistics Norway (2020b), in 2019, 40.7 per cent of the ECC staff consisted of pre-school teachers. The OECD (Engel et al, 2015) has previously criticised Norway for having unskilled staff that work with children without being supervised by pedagogically educated staff. Since 2018, the law has regulated the ratio between staff (non-skilled and skilled) and the number of children for all ECCs. For children aged 0–3, this ratio is 1:3, and for children aged 3–6, the ratio is 1:6 (The Norwegian Directorate of Education and Training, 2020). There is a general lack of skilled staff in many OECD countries, and many countries face recruitment challenges in regard to skilled staff, including Finland and Sweden (OECD, 2019). In Denmark, statistics show that in 2014 an average staff–child ratio was 3.5 children (0–3 years) per full-time staff member, and 6.8 children per staff member for children aged from 3 to 6 years. There have been staff reductions over the last ten years, which have resulted in a decrease in staff–child ratios. There are also substantial differences in the staff–child ratios among the 98 municipalities in Denmark (Schreyer and Oberhuemer, 2017a). Sweden has no recommendations for staff–child ratios, but Skolverket suggests group sizes of 6 to 12 children for the ages of 1–3 years, and 9 to 15 children for the ages 4–5 years. National statistics from Sweden suggest a staff–child ratio of 5.2 children per staff member in pre-schools and 16.4 children per staff member in pre-school classes (Schreyer and Oberhuemer, 2017b).

Time in work organisations

In the modern organisation, the coordination of work tasks rests on the possibility of dividing time in sequences, for example, measuring time and selling time. Adam (2002) relates clock time to a modern industrial economic logic of production. Central to national work time regimes are regulations of work time: the standardisation of the duration of the working day and the right to lunchtime breaks. This applies to Norwegian ECCs. Clock time and calendars regulate the activities at the centres, such as daily meals and weekly field trips. This reflects some facets of the rhythm of the organisation. This rhythm mirrors the tempo of the work. It can also be the object of temporal shifts if workflows are altered or interrupted by events (Staudenmayer et al, 2002). If one assistant leaves the group, this might generate a temporal shift that intensifies the work for others.

Efficiency measures have marked organisations since the 1970s and are central to New Public Management ideas (Radnor et al, 2012). The efficient use of work time in organisations is particularly inspired by lean management principles, with a widespread impact on private and public organisations (Carter et al, 2013; Bortolotti et al, 2015). Lean-management aims to reduce all kinds of waste and slack in production. Efficiency measures to reduce slack produce *meagre organisations*, who have a scarcity of resources compared to their assigned tasks (Trägårdh and Lindberg, 2004). In a meagre organisation, one could expect rhythms marked by high tempos with little possibility to slow down.

Time and care in organisations

Caring consists of activities that 'include everything we do to maintain, continue and repair our world so that we can live in it as well as possible' (Fisher and Tronto, 1990: 40). Adam (2002) loosely classifies every human practice that is dependent on context and matter as care. Fisher and Tronto (1990) point to time as an enabling factor for caring. Care takes the time that it takes; it is context-bound and follows a relational logic focused on the needs of others. Care is a central form of human action and is related to interpersonal virtues associated with private relationships such as 'compassion, attentiveness, empathy, and attention to detail' (Sevenhuijsen, 1998: 5).

The temporal logic of caring can collide with organisational time logic. Organisations must divide tasks and organise them with a start and end in clock time, whereas caring must answer to a constant flow of others' needs. Consequently, ECCs are potential 'battlefields' of different time logics and this might explain the social-reproductive contradiction of organisations pointed to by Fraser (2016). Adam (2002: 23) argues that the problem of reconciling paid work and care in families facing an industrial time logic has created 'a shadowland' of work and re/production in which the world's women live. This chapter explores this 'shadowland' in potential meagre ECC organisational frame and in situations where new tasks, such as competence-raising schemes to meet quality demands, are introduced to leaders and staff responsible for caring. Tufte and Dahl (2016) find that Danish care workers in the home–care sector produce different time-navigating practices to handle conflicting time logics, such as figuratively leaving time outside while practising care, practising individualised routinisation, multitasking and postponing. However, the authors do not discuss leadership.

The metaphor of orchestrating describes leading in time. Orchestration refers to the arrangement of different tasks in time, while trying to influence performance, duration, interplay and tempo; and it enables us to see more clearly the role of leadership. On an organisational level, however, Adam (2002) argues that the compression and intensification of processes are key aims in the quest for time control and the achievement of efficiency, which is likely to be present in meagre organisations. Returning to Adam's notion of the shadowland of work and reproduction, this shadowland might exist in meagre organisations and appears when caring is practised within the temporal logic of the organisation. Previous research suggests that organisations handle the care crisis by tight orchestration and high tempo. Thus, I ask the following questions:

• How do ECC leaders and staff experience the shadowland of organisational reproduction work when taking part in part in ECC competence-raising schemes and measures?
• Are there traces of time strategies among leaders and staff who handle care and competence raising, and what are the preconditions for these strategies to work?

Method

To shed light on the research questions, I analyse qualitative interview data gathered from staff members and managers on their experiences with 'in-house' ECC competence building. The material consists of two sets of qualitative data from seven ECCs, representing the cases involved in this study (Yin, 2018).

The first dataset explores how students and staff experience work-based early childhood teacher education (ECTE). ECTE consists of a bachelor's degree in ECEC teaching and is obtained through a four-year education. It differs from regular pre-school teacher education by requiring student employment in an ECC during the education process. Students have to work minimum 20 per cent or maximum 50 per cent in an ECC during education. In ECTE, the ECC organisation is supposed to play a central role in the student's training, and the staff is supposed to learn from, and together with, the student (Ministry of Education and Research, 2017a). One assumption is that the staff as a whole will benefit from the student's learning, which will raise the overall ECEC quality. This dataset consists of three ECCs that host and employ an ECTE student. Representatives from the staff and the students were interviewed. Documents and visits to the ECC centre supplement the interview data. In this chapter, cases 1–3 are ECTE cases.

The second dataset explores competence-raising measures in ECCs organised according to the principles of ECC-based competence raising, as defined in the National Strategy for Competence and Recruitment in Norwegian ECCs (Ministry of Education and Research, 2017a). Accordingly, competence shall be raised among all staff groups through work-based processes, including external competence suppliers (for example, universities). The selection criteria were that ECCs organised such competence raising in local or regional networks. They represented a variety of work-based schemes and ownership. In just one of the schemes, the ECC had the project funding to hire a substitute. In the network dataset, representatives for all staff groups were interviewed. In this chapter, cases 4–7 are ECC-based competence-raising cases. Cases 6 and 7 belong to the same competence-raising network.

The interview guides include the experiences of the informants concerning 'in-house' training, organisation and leading; thus, they are well suited to shed light on the chapter's research questions. Recording the interviews ensured reliability. All the interviews were transcribed verbatim in the network dataset. All the director and student interviews were transcribed verbatim in the ECTE dataset, whereas the interviews with other staff members were summed up in written reports that refer to minutes and seconds found in the audio files. Particularly relevant sections of the group interviews regarding caring were transcribed verbatim. Table 9.1 provides an overview of some characteristics of the datasets.

Data were analysed using NVivo and followed a theme-based approach (Brinkman and Kvale, 2015). During the analysis process, the issue between time and time to care appeared striking in the material and thus is further explored. The small size of the sample prevents the possibility to draw general conclusions about orchestrating a care–centred rhythm. The external validity

Table 9.1: Overview of ECCs by number, competence measure scheme, ownership and number of informants

ECC (case)	Main theme for competence measure	Number of informants
1	ECTE	7
2	ECTE	5
3	ECTE	4
4	Network/ECC-based	4
5	Network/ECC-based	3
6	Network/ECC-based	3
7	Network/ECC-based	3
	Number of informants:	29

was low, but the analytical validity was strengthened by blind review and the presentation of drafts in a project group.

The research project was approved by the data protection official for research and was conducted in accordance with the ethical guidelines for research complied by the Norwegian National Research Ethics Committees.

Result

Child-centredness

All the participants expressed a common appreciation for their work in the ECC and a motivation to better the lives of the children. They prepared a meaningful everyday life for the children. I interpret this as an expression of a prevailing child–centredness among the staff that underscores the value of tending to children's needs. It expresses a relational logic founded upon the needs of others (Fisher and Tronto, 1990). The relational logic and child-centredness works as the source of meaning participants use to rationalise their actions and practices.

There are several aspects to this relational logic, which relates strongly to caring as an attitude directed to answer to the needs of others (Sevenhuijsen, 1998). One assistant, in case 4, stressed that the most important ability to do a good job was "to be able to understand the needs of others, first and foremost the children's needs". An assistant in case 5 replied that she valued play and friendship but that "most important is how you meet the children and care for them. Of course, this is also true for parents and colleagues—how we shall work together. However, the children are the most important".

The data suggest that this child-centredness is connected to the here and now – the (well-)being of children – such as their play, relations and friendships. This resonates with Fisher and Tronto's definition of care as an activity aimed at living 'as well as possible' (1990: 49). However, this also includes considerations for fellow co–workers and parents and the feeling of responsibility for the children's welfare. The staff represent several caring relationships. Even though they stress that children are prioritised, this might entail crossing interests, where a wage–earner mentality is set in motion, for example, a staff orientation towards the worker collective (Lysgaard and Kalleberg, 2001). Several managers in both datasets note that it is a central leadership task to turn the staff's attention to child-centredness. An example is a manager who stresses that the activities shall be meaningful for the children, and not necessarily done because they are convenient for the staff.

Caring is also seen as superior to learning, where learning becomes a mediator for caring in terms of building and maintaining the children's well-being (Fisher and Tronto, 1990). One of the assistants exemplified this by using learning situations to build good self-esteem: "For me, it is not important that children start school as masters in drawing, but that they develop good self-esteem, whether it is while getting dressed, in doing art and so on" (assistant, single interview, case 5). In contrast to families, ECCs are pedagogical undertakings with a specified societal mandate that includes caring, learning and play. Professional perspectives and standards are evident in the material. This also connects to a relational logic. Here, care is approached as one of several aspects of professional practice. Although professional practice in the ECC is based on care and good interpersonal relations, some of the staff, particularly formally educated staff, underscored that the organisation had to be a professional, pedagogical institution. This implies a practice that is different to merely caring. Stronger attention to pedagogy was described as increasing over time by one assistant who stated that "it is not only caring anymore". She had worked for decades in ECEC and felt pressured to take part in competence-raising schemes and pay more attention to pedagogy. On this background we can interpret the ECCs as the shadowland described by Adam (2002). It is imprinted by a strong relational logic and child-centredness that can be associated with a temporal logic of care.

Daily rhythm and tempo of the ECCs

The so-called 'daily rhythm' often organises the ECC activities. Case 3 described this rhythm for the parents in an information leaflet and it divided the day into 11 sequences. For example, adult-organised activities start at 9.30 am, because most of the children have arrived by that time. At 10.30 am, there is an assembly before lunch, which is at 11.00 am. This daily rhythm illustrates the organisational time logic at work.

Several informants described their workday as hectic. This indicates labour-intensiveness due to a steady flow of tasks. The staff must be present and available for the children at all times since the children cannot tend to themselves. There are few breaks described apart from lunchbreaks. For the ECTE students, the ECC is supposed to be an important learning arena during their education. However, the tempo of the work makes it hard for this student to reflect on the practice undertaken in the work situation: "Everyday life consists of a lot of practical stuff. During the day, this and that shall be done. It is more than expected if you can have 5 minutes to reflect over situations during the day" (ECTE student, case 3). The director in case 3 problematised that they had challenges with regard to facilitating mutual learning between the ECE student and the staff due to time pressure in the ECC. The director of case 6 stated that the tempo was high and that no one could lurk around idly because they were dependent on all the staff being present. She described the ECEC sector as a tough trade with a high sick-leave rate: "Of course, it is always high pressure."

This does not necessarily reflect a hectic day for the children. The director in case 4 underscored that the staff had to adjust their working rhythm so that the activity flow and rhythm of the children's activities should not be disrupted by the staff's lunchbreaks. She considered the staff's break as an event that broke up the natural flow of the children's daily activities. They regularly go on walks in the local environment, during which the staff do not have a break until they return. The staff breaks are postponed to ensure the occurrence of what is by perceived the director as a natural flow:

> 'When it comes to how we organise the day, we always think how we shall arrange the day; we are open for 9 hours, and these hours must be used in the best possible way for the children. We always have to think that this shall be good for the children, first thing.'

She compared the everyday life in the ECEC with the hectic everyday life of families and she wanted her ECC to be a place for children to experience having ample time and a slow tempo. Thus, the staff, encouraged by leaders, put the children's interests first, trying to spare them the effects of the rapid pace. Sheltering children from the effects of the organisational time logic is one way the staff try to handle social-reproductive contradictions in the organisation. Staff put individual needs to the side. This process contributes to constituting the shadowland of work/reproduction that characterises the care crisis (Fraser, 2016) in meagre ECCs. Organisations marked by a high tempo and child-centredness shall embark on ECC-based competence-raising schemes.

Competence raising as a mixed blessing

Staff members are ambivalent when facing ECEC-based competence measures. They described a wide variety of measures. On the one hand, the staff value them as necessary and positive. The pedagogical leader in case 5 felt that a common competence-raising scheme involving all the staff had positive effects that made it easier to work together collectively: "The practice becomes more equal, and we as a staff group get insights into each other's understandings."

Staff members were motivated to raise the competence level when they observed the direct positive effects of competence-raising schemes for the individual child. The relational and caring logic affects the assessment of competence-raising schemes. For example, one assistant in case 1 underscored that participating in the guidance had developed her self-reflection, empathy, care and raised her amelioration of relational aspects of the work. In this respect, the staff welcome competence-raising projects as measures for raising quality.

On the other hand, there was also a scepticism against such schemes because they could represent disruptions in the work rhythm by making staff members periodically leave the unit. This would potentially represent a temporal shift and increase the work intensity for the remaining staff and were seen as negative for both the children and their colleagues. One skilled assistant in case 7 stated: "I think the everyday life in the ECEC can be pretty hectic; therefore, I rather quickly question things that can take our time away from the children. But when I see results, that it is a good project, that motivates me."

Case 5 was unique in experiencing a competence-raising project that financed substitutes. However, this proved problematic. One assistant observed that substitutes challenged the continuity in staff, on which the youngest children depend. Others who did not have substitutes felt guilty when they left their colleagues alone in the department, knowing that they would have a more stressful time at work. Some assistants had experienced work intensification because their colleagues had left for guidance. This indicates a conflict of interest between taking part in schemes that feel necessary but put colleagues in a possibly difficult situation. Such feelings express a solidarity in the working collective. Schemes that take staff members out of their department seem to produce temporal challenges. Such schemes can become time thieves that potentially generate time shifts. Higher levels of work intensity are perceived as negative for the everyday life of both children and staff. One of the directors summed up this issue as follows: "Time is detrimental in an ECC because we have children here at all times, and that binds us. It is difficult to have a long-term perspective on development work or raising competence. To be together, working together as a group to raise competence, is very time-consuming" (director, case 6). This supports an interpretation of ECCs as potential meagre organisations, where the staff is set to meet the needs of children following a temporal logic of care. However, there seems to be little 'slack' in the organisation that can be used for competence raising. In such a situation, staff members find themselves in the shadowland of work/ reproduction in the ECCs when they have to care for children and raise their competence under a high work tempo. They experience this as an ambivalent place to be in, one that is marked by feelings of joy, guilt and scepticism. We shall now see how the directors try to organise the organisational rhythm to handle the task of raising competence while at the same act according to a relational logic founded upon the needs of the children.

Leaders' temporal orchestration in the shadowland of work and reproduction

The described organisational processes create a shadowland *of work and re/ production* that the ECC staff dwell in. The next section explores how leaders orchestrate centre-based competence against this backdrop.

Recycling old rhythms or creating new?

The most common way of handling this situation is to use the existing meeting structure of the centres, where the directors try to 'recycle' and reorganise in the endeavour to raise competence and become learning organisations. To pursue the orchestrating metaphor, they continue with the same meeting rhythm but follow a different tune.

In some centres leaders guide and counsel staff during staff meetings. For example, ECTE students use the meetings to become informed about the themes or practices learned in their education. The unit meetings are often once a week and described as lasting for approximately one hour. However, the staff members also need to use these meetings to organise their pedagogical work and discuss the children's groups. They can be held in the afternoon, when the children have left the facility, but this presupposes the use of overtime or taking time off in lieu of salary. The director in case 6 reported facilitating meetings in the afternoon and evenings to carry out the reflection work needed to follow up on an ECC-based competence-raising scheme. She compensated for this with an overtime salary, thereby enabling them more work-time flexibility: "We only have the one meeting in the afternoon and 5 planning days a year. We can have one pedagogical leader meeting and one unit meeting a week. In the unit meeting, we collaborate so that we are taking care of each other's children."

In personnel meetings and on planning days, the staff group meets as a whole. The personnel meetings take place every second or third week or once a month in these ECCs. In some cases, they are arranged to take place after the centre's closing time to not affect the time spent with the children. In case 4, the participants recounted their ongoing competence development work related to their participation in a regional competence network. There is a long tradition of having planning days in Norwegian ECCs, during which children stay at home. In regard to this type of material, they are, for the most part, used not for planning but for competence raising. The network gatherings are always arranged during the planning days. The participants particularly mention the planning days because during such days, the centres are closed and, thus, the children do not notice their participation in the competence schemes.

The directors preferred schemes and measures that could be implemented within existing organisational structures. They hesitate to enter into projects where staff are required to leave the unit. The directors assess projects and schemes by how time-consuming they are. If a scheme is regarded as too time-consuming, she might reject it. In reflecting on the time used by ECTE students in case 1, the director was critical of this arrangement because she felt that the students had demanded too much time for guidance outside of the existing meeting structure. In cases 6 and 7, the ECCs also applied a commercialised and very structured system that was easy to learn. This system presented ready-made templates that explained the steps in the guiding process. This made it effective to use.

The ECEC workers do not problematise this 'recycling' of the meeting structure with competence raising. Nevertheless, the director in case 6 mentioned that this way of using the meeting structure superseded other tasks: "it becomes too little time to work with other things, such as health, environment, and safety (HES) issues". She also stated that if there were too many projects going on, she often postponed some of them.

This leadership practice of not altering the rhythm but rather resetting the tune is evident in the leader's stressing of the meeting content. One of the directors stated that she had become very strict in her meeting leadership style. She did not tolerate small talk and discussions on very practical issues in the personnel meetings. Strong meeting discipline includes an expectation of staff to be prepared for guiding sessions. Directors also singled out other tasks they assessed as being superfluous or taking unnecessary time away for the children. One example given was that of refusing to use time for language assessing all the children. Such gatekeeping of tasks, therefore, becomes part of the time orchestration of leaders in the shadowland of reproduction/work. In summary, they reduce the amount of 'slack' available and make the organisation further efficient.

There are, however, some examples related to the material of leaders when altering the organisational rhythm to facilitate competence development. One director stated:

'It is in a way hopeless because I know they are very busy. They have 8 hours, after which they have had enough of the children. So, I have to prepare for them to be able to make it. For example, I say to them that we only take 6 hours from this day, so that you can have time to read, or we use half an hour to read an article in the meeting and then talk about it. Or they can work a bit longer and then later take the time off.' (Director, case 6)

In these ways, she gave time to the staff. A rarer strategy was to give unskilled assistants some time to plan activities. Having budgetary room for this was, however, a premise. I also found that the staff themselves are willing to help each other take on more tasks so that their colleagues can participate in competence-raising projects as a way of sharing the time burden.

Filling the time gaps

The directors and staff urge the raising of competence without taking staff away from the children. To be able to do this, they actively use informal and short meetings with staff, for example, to obtain information on competence needs and wishes of the staff group, instead of using time to make staff members fill in competence-measuring templates. The director in case 4 stated that "it is my leadership style, I think, walking around and watching them and asking them". Regarding working in a 'here-and-now' manner, guidance was also described by a pedagogical leader in case 5 as follows:

'A lot of things one has to deal with here and now, also because of the time pressure. There are no possibilities to sit down and discuss the happening, [jokingly] even though that would be the ideal, to have a substitute sitting here waiting to step in when we needed to talk together. Well, no.'

By guiding colleagues in such a here-and-now manner, the directors do not risk interrupting the workflow. The staff fills in small pockets of 'empty' time, such as periods of the day when the children sleep or before they go on their lunchbreak, to have informal reflections and discussions together. Another strategy is to bring the children with them on activities that are also part of competence raising. This is the case with the ECTE students who do student tasks together with the children. The director in case 1 said, "You have to use everyday life. That is the time we have available. It becomes a flow of children and adults in the way we work." These are forms of multitasking. The result is intensifying the work rhythm. As such, the orchestration of time and organisational rhythms are a mechanism that reproduces and upholds the shadowland of reproduction/work in these organisations.

Preparing the 'orchestra'

Finally, the leaders are also working on time orchestration by preparing and motivating 'the orchestra', namely the staff group, to take on the task of raising their competence in a situation of high work intensity. They do this by making competence schemes and projects meaningful for the staff. For example, they define where staff shall focus their attention during a hectic day, as stated by the director in case 7: "My role, is to be the one who says, 'Now we will have to focus on this and use our time on this', to arrange for that." It also entails discussing the feeling of guilt that leaving the children seems to cause in some and arguing for the necessity of it. The director in case 5 related this to a female-dominated staff group as well as parental attitudes:

'In our centre, we are all women, and it is a female-dominated sector. Maybe they carry a guilty consciousness due to a lacking professional awareness. When we have such meetings, it is for a reason. It is to become better and to act more professionally. It can be marked by an attitude of "but then we are away from the children". And it is the same as the parents. They also say, "We chose your centre because we know there are few meetings here, you are much more present with the children here".'

Here, we see that the director is negotiating the downsides of the relational logic by asking if leaving the children is an expression of lacking professionalism. The directors also employed top-down decisions to participate in the project by using success stories of others and professional arguments to make sense of the project for the staff group. Others described bottom-up approaches, claiming it was the best way to motivate the staff to take on competence raising. This was, for example, undertaken by involving staff in planning processes and buying books, as related by the director in case 1. She also worked hard to establish and maintain a learning culture that enabled using situations in everyday life for collective learning and thereby 'filling the gaps'. This included being very explicit about the professional values and themes to which they were supposed to relate the everyday discussions. She underscored the role of building trust among the staff in that regard; this could be to find an individual's field of interest and be open to staff members discussing their own competence needs. It is also about making the demand posed by the organisational learning culture clear for the individual employee. The director in case 4 stated:

'We have been very explicit in saying that if you are not interested, of course with a dash of humour, then we are sure that there is a job waiting for you down there, as we point to the nearest gas station. So, you know there are other possibilities if you have no wish to take part in the learning culture here.'

Leading to prepare the orchestra entails moulding the mindset and feelings of the staff group. It is also about communicating demands and creating images of what it takes to be a relevant and good employee, as evident in this quote. It is about 'developing staff who can lead themselves', as stated by one director. In these processes, a relational logic of care becomes important, as it appeals to worker motivation to make the staff endure dwelling in the shadowland of work and care.

Conclusion

This chapter explored the care crisis (Fraser, 2016) in Norwegian ECCs and how it is experienced and handled by staff members that face competence-raising measures in the name of quality. The preoccupation with quality in education has been related to neoliberal governing rationalities (Hunkin, 2018). We find traces of the care crisis in Norwegian ECCs by exploring the 'shadowland' of work and care. There is a strong relational logic prevalent in the data. It values the moral aspects of caring and puts children at the centre of attention. The staff highly values the here-and-now perspective of children's everyday lives and does not necessarily pay attention to how the ECC represents an investment in children's lives, as underscored in a neoliberal discourse. It follows a temporal logic of care; it takes the time it takes. The temporal logic of care is realised within the frames of the meager organisation. Almost all the interviewees discussed working days in a high tempo setting and recounted responding to the constant need of children – with little slack and few breaks. Together, these two aspects add up to a contradiction between care and work that constitutes the shadowland of re/production in which they dwell. Still, the staff members must embark on ECC-based competence-raising schemes introduced by the government to increase the level of care and teaching quality. The relational logic is used to assess the value of the schemes, although they might represent work intensification and a faster work tempo.

Leaders apply a range of temporal leadership strategies to implement ECC-based competence measure schemes. They help orchestrate the competence-raising process within the industrial time frames of the meagre organisation. Time organisation is 'engineered', and the directors implement the schemes within the existing temporal structure of the organisation by recycling the organisational structure or by filling time gaps. Temporal strategies familiar with other studies, such as multitasking and postponing tasks, are applied (Tufte and Dahl, 2016). Work intensification becomes a result of these strategies. The directors also work on the mindset of the staff to motivate and make sense of the competence schemes. They actively argue from a child-centred and relational logic to urge the staff to take on the extra workload and take part in the ECC learning cultures. Only seldom is the capacity altered in the form of adding new resources.

ECCs as organisations strive to answer the needs of children. As seen in other studies (Vike, 2004), ECC employees are set to realise the goals of the welfare state. They are forced to handle the care crisis produced by meagre organisations. The relational and child-centred logic, therefore, becomes central in the creation of an organisational, temporal and attitudinal 'firewall' that protects the children from the strains placed on the organisation caused by the reproductive contradiction produced by the organisation's surroundings. The same logic motivates the staff to shoulder a more intensive workday. At first glance, such a child-centred relational logic and valuation of caring reflects supportable Nordic ECEC values. However, there are some dangers to this approach. It urges staff to place their own interests second and cultivate child–staff relationships for the best interest of the child. A possible effect of this approach is that the capitalist aspect of being hired and paid is toned down and the corporate non-responsibilty towards staff's need to reproduce its labour power is harder to detect. One might understand this as a caring paradox in organisations: the goal rational application of a relational logic founded on the need of others can actually undermine the organisation's ability to care for its staff. Staff are recruited into the child-centred project as an individual calling. Such individualisation of responsibility is in line with previous findings from Denmark by Monrad (2017), who showed that it becomes harder to argue for workers' rights and to point the finger at structural capacity issues. One might ask what protects the staff from the reproductive contradiction and bring them out of the shadowland? Compared to other Nordic countries, Norway spends relatively more resources on ECEC (Engel et al, 2015); thus, one might assume that such a care crisis can also be found in other Nordic ECCs. This should be further explored. Maybe the solution to the care crisis is found in another characteristic of the Nordic welfare state, such as the tripartite collaborations and the strong unions? Making the care crisis a capacity problem and an issue for the worker collective, rather than making it a motivational and leadership issue, might bring it from the shadowland and into the light.

References

Acker, J. (2006) *Class Questions: Feminist Answers*, Lanham: Rowman & Littlefield.

Adam, B. (2002) 'The gendered time politics of globalization: Of shadowlands and elusive justice', *Feminist Review*, 70(1): 3–29.

Aslanian, T.K. (2017) 'Ready or not, here they come! Care as a material and organizational practice in ECEC for children under two', *Global Studies of Childhood*, 7(4): 323–334.

Bortolotti, T., Boscari, S. and Danese, P. (2015) 'Successful lean implementation: Organizational culture and soft lean practices', *International Journal of Production Economics*, 160: 182–201.

Brinkman, S. and Kvale, S. (2015) *InterViews: Learning the Craft of Qualitative Research Interviewing* (3rd edn), London: SAGE.

Carter, B., Danford, A., Howcroft, D., Richardson, H., Smith, A. and Taylor, P. (2013) ' "Stressed out of my box": Employee experience of lean working and occupational ill-health in clerical work in the UK public sector', *Work, Employment & Society*, 27(5): 747–767.

Eidevald, C. and Engdahl, I. (2018) *Utbilding och undervisning i förskolan. Omsorgsfullt och lekfullt stöd för lärande och utveckling*, Stockholm: Liber.

Enehaug, H., Gamperiene, M. and Grimsmo, A. (2008) *Arbeidsmiljøet i barnehagen: en casestudie i 4 barnehager i offentlig og privat sektor*, Oslo: Arbeidsforskningsinstituttet.

Engel, A., Barnett, W.S., Anders, Y. and Taguma, M. (2015) *Early Childhood Education and Care Policy Review: Norway*. Paris: OECD.

Fisher, B. and Tronto, J. (1990) 'Towards a feminist theory of caring' in E. Abel and M. Nelson (eds) *Circles of Care: Work and Identity in Women's Lives*, New York: State University of New York Press, pp 35–62.

Fraser, N. (2016) 'Contradictions of capital and care', *New Left Review*, 100: 99–117.

Haugset, A.S. (2018) 'Institusjonelt eiermangfold og et likeverdig barnehagetilbud', *Nordisk barnehageforskning*, 17(1): 1–14.

Hunkin, E. (2018) 'Whose quality? The (mis)uses of quality reform in early childhood and education policy', *Journal of Education Policy*, 33(4): 443–456.

Karila, K. (2012) 'A Nordic perspective on early childhood education and care policy', *European Journal of Education*, 47(4): 584–595.

Ljunggren, B. and Lauritzen, T. (2018) 'Likestillingsintegrering i kvinnedominerte sektorer – horisontale styringsutfordringer', *Tidsskrift for samfunnsforskning*, 59(2): 157–179.

Ljunggren, B., Moen, K.H., Monica, S., Naper, L.R., Fagerholt, R.A., Leirset, E. and Gotvassli, K.Å. (2017) *Barnehagens rammeplan mellom styring og skjønn- en kunnskapsstatus om implementering og gjennomføring med videre anbefalinger*, 2/2017, Trondheim: DMMH.

Lysgaard, S. and Kalleberg, R. (2001) *Arbeiderkollektivet: en studie i de underordnedes sosiologi* (3rd edn), Oslo: Universitetsforlaget.

Ministry of Education and Research (2011) *Rammeplan for barnehagens innhold og oppgaver*, Oslo: Ministry of Education and Research.

Ministry of Education and Research (2017a) *Framework Plan for Kindergartens*, Oslo: Ministry of Education and Research.

Ministry of Education and Research (2017b) *Kompetanse for fremtidens barnehage. Revidert strategi for kompetanse og rekruttering 2018–2022* [online]. Oslo: Ministry of Education and Research. Available from: https://www.regjeringen.no [accessed 28 June 2017].

Monrad, M. (2017) 'Emotional labour and governmentality: Productive power in childcare', *Contemporary Issues in Early Childhood*, 18(3): 281–293.

Nicolaisen, H., Seip, Å.A. and Jordfald, B. (2012) *Tidstyver i barnehagen: tidsbruk i barnehager i bydel Alna* [online]. FAFO-rapport, no 01/2012. Available from: https://www.fafo.no/media/com_netsukii/20228.pdf [accessed 4 March 2020].

The Nowegian Directorate of Education and Training (2020) *Bemanningsnorm og skjerpet pedagognorm – hvordan ligger barnehagene an?* Statistikknotat 4/2018 [online]. The Norwegian Directorate of Education and Training. Available from: https://www.udir.no/tall-og-forskning/finn-forskning/tema/Statistikknotat-bemanningsnorm-barnehage/ [accessed 22 November 2020].

OECD (2019) *Good Practice for Good Jobs in Early Childhood Education and Care* [online]. Available from: https://www.oecd-ilibrary.org/content/publication/64562be6-en [accessed 27 March 2020].

Radnor, Z.J., Holweg, M. and Waring, J. (2012) 'Lean in healthcare: The unfilled promise?', *Social Science & Medicine*, 74(3): 364–371.

Schreyer, I. and Oberhuemer, P. (2017a) 'Denmark: Key contextual data' in P. Oberhuemer and I. Schreyer (eds) *Workforce Profiles in Systems of Early Childhood Education and Care in Europe* [online]. Available from: www.seepro.eu/English/Country_Reports.htm [accessed 28 June 2021]

Schreyer, I. and Oberhuemer, P. (2017b) 'Sweden: Key contextual data' in P. Oberhuemer and I. Schreyer (eds) *Workforce Profiles in Systems of Early Childhood Education and Care in Europe* [online]. Available from: www.seepro.eu/English/Country_Reports.htm [accessed 28 June 2021]

Segerholm, C. (2012) 'The quality turn', *Education Inquiry*, 3(2): 115–122.

Sevenhuijsen, S. (1998) *Citizenship and the Ethics of Care: Feminist Considerations of Justice, Morality and Politics*, London: Routledge.

Staudenmayer, N., Tyre, M. and Perlow, L. (2002) 'Time to change: Temporal shifts as enablers of organizational change', *Organization Science*, 13(5): 583–597.

Statistics Norway (2020a) *Table 3: Children in Kindergartens by Hours of Attendance and Different Age Groups*. [Online]. Statistics Norway. Available from: http://www https://www.ssb.no/en/utdanning/statistikker/barnehager [accessed 22 November 2020].

Statistics Norway (2020b) *Kindergartens. 12562: Selected Key Figures Kindergartens (M) 2015 – 2019*. [Online]. Statistics Norway. Available from: https://www.ssb.no/statbank/table/12562/tableViewLayout1/ [accessed 22 November 2020].

Trägårdh, B. and Lindberg, K. (2004) 'Curing a meagre health care system by lean methods: Translating "chains of care" in the Swedish health care sector', *The International Journal of Health Planning and Management*, 19(4): 383–398.

Tufte, P. and Dahl, H.M. (2016) 'Navigating the field of temporally framed care in the Danish home care sector', *Sociology of Health & Illness*, 38(1): 109–122.

Vike, H. (2004) *Velferd uten grenser: den norske velferdsstaten ved veiskillet*, Oslo: Akribe.

Yin, R.K. (2018) *Case Study Research and Applications: Design and Methods* (6th edn), Los Angeles: SAGE.

10

Conclusion: Less caring and less gender-equal Nordic states

Lise Lotte Hansen and Hanne Marlene Dahl

This book began by asking whether it is justified to talk about the existence of a care crisis in the Nordic welfare states that have implemented neoliberal reforms and, if so, what are the characteristics of this crisis and the major areas of concern in terms of gender equality and welfare state sustainability? The book concludes that it is possible to talk about a care crisis in the Nordic welfare states, and that there are issues of concern regarding both gender equality and welfare state sustainability. It is an uneven crisis, which takes different forms in the various fields of care and in the different Nordic states. Although the care crisis might not be fully visible yet, it produces insufficient and inadequate care, sometimes poor working conditions and too little time for the care workers to care for themselves, their families and communities. However, the Nordic welfare states have also made a difference to the depth of the crisis: regulations and institutions have prevented the development of a full crisis. Moreover, care workers, care-givers and care-receivers and their organisations are taking part in social struggles against the consequences of neoliberalism and financialisation. Yet, the outcome has – so far – been less caring and less gender-equal Nordic states.

What is a care crisis?

In the introduction, we argued in favour of rethinking the notion of a care crisis. We defined a care crisis as characterised by inadequate resources for care and the absence of 'good-enough care', applying the theorisations of Hochschild (1995) and Fraser (2016) and combining them with the insights of Phillips (1994) considering the industries of care. In this book, the contributors have directed their attention to what happens *inside* the Nordic welfare state(s). Resources refer to money, time and the labour force: A care crisis is not exclusively constituted by recruitment problems, although these often occur as a symptom of a crisis of care.

Three of the chapters discuss in detail how the care crisis should be understood and which issues in particular should be highlighted. Dahl (Chapter 2) pointed out that the discourse(s) and conceptualisations of the care crisis in the international literature silence what constitutes good care, the complex identity of care-givers and care-receivers, and elder care (in opposition to childcare). Moreover, professional care and the extended, positive role of fathers are neglected. In the Nordic context, she argued that unpaid care work in particular is silenced. Kovalainen (Chapter 4) also highlighted how unpaid care work has been lacking in (feminist) research, despite the 'substantial contribution to most countries' economics as well as to individual and social wellbeing'. Her most important point is that technology turns into *the* remedy to solve the care crisis, a remedy which ignores the complexity of the care crisis as well as the need for care in real interactions (as opposed to virtual).

In Chapter 3, Hansen, Bjørnholt and Horn developed a model of care crisis dynamics based on Nancy Fraser's care crisis theory by extending and restating her theorisation, and they discussed examples of these dynamics in Denmark and Norway. They identified several care crisis indicators within the following five dimensions: fundamental dynamics in capitalist societies, market, state, civil society and gender equality. These indicators concern a wide range of ways that the care crisis surfaces in Denmark and Norway. Examples include increasing financialisation, privatisation and commercialisation of care provision; a less social-democratic state and a more neoliberal and social investment state; a dual-earner–dual-carer model with less involvement of the state and more responsibilities for care left to families; and an increasing focus on fathering and men's equality with less status given to mothering. However, another indicator is how the crisis leads to resistance and social struggles. This highlights the dynamic and contradictory nature of the care crisis in the Nordic welfare states, which will be elaborated in the next sections.

The complexity of the care crisis

In Chapter 2, Dahl demonstrated the need to be reflexive about travelling and analytical notions and to rethink them as context-sensitive concepts. The discussion at the beginning of the book examined the care crisis concept in context and argued that case studies of selected areas would provide a deeper understanding of the care crisis. This is evident in the contributions in this book. The depth and extent of the care crisis become visible by focusing on micro processes in everyday practices. Also apparent is the complexity, and partly contradictory nature, of the crisis. Relating macro discourses to everyday practices of care provides a deeper understanding of how neoliberalism impacts the reframing of care, thereby changing the way in which care is provided in care practices. Neoliberalism reframes care into a 'thinner' form of care, omitting elements of care, stressing the self-responsibilising of the recipient of care (Dahl, 2012), and governing care more intensively and in more standardised ways. Increased governance means an increase in the cross-pressures experienced by care professionals and care workers. These cross-pressures are not identical to those described by US political scientist Michael Lipsky (1980), which arise between the resources available and the demands of clients/citizens. Instead, cross-pressures are increasingly between the many conflicting ideals and values *within* the state and the governance of care.

The contributions in this book raise a number of cross-cutting issues, such as what constitutes good care, working conditions, and caring on market terms.

Discussions about *good care* – and *good-enough care* (Williams, 2001) – and how to achieve it refer to care work conditions, the qualifications of care professionals, and problems in professional, managed and bureaucratised care. Management strategies, service ideologies and constant restructuring of the work reduce the possibility to give good – or good-enough – care. Instead, it is left to the individual care worker to make up for this, often with severe consequences both for the care worker (breakdowns, mental and physical pain) and the care recipient (mistreatment and neglect). The quality of care is also about misrecognition of existing professional skills and re-articulating them in new ideals of the good, care professional, and about 'unlearning' educational qualifications brought forward by neoliberalism (see Chapters 5, 7, 8 and 9). However, discussions on good care have to include how technologies transform ideals of care; instead of supporting care values, they 'set the value standards *for* care' (see Chapter 4). These problems are connected closely to problems with *working conditions*. A takeaway from the chapters is the overload of professional carers' tasks. In kindergartens, hospitals and elder care, professionals are struggling to make ends meet in the allotted time. Pedagogues struggle to care for children and to find the time to develop their analytical and caring competences, whereas nurses and professionals in elder care are increasingly physically, emotionally and mentally exhausted (see Chapters 5, 7, 8 and 9). Physical, emotional and mental exhaustion is also present among cleaners (see Chapter 3). Professionals struggle to reduce cross-pressures and avoid burnout. In elder care in Finland and Sweden, care professionals experience a fast work pace, exhaustion and a fear of 'forgetting things', which sometimes results in care failures. Care professionals experience moral distress due to not being able to provide the necessary – and good-enough – care. Experiences like these tend to become part of a vicious circle. Understaffing/staff shortages and a governance of details[1] can feed into processes of mental, emotional and physical exhaustion. These might lead to early retirement, which again might result in staff shortages and increasing work pressure and illness for the professional carers left behind. This becomes a vicious circle as it tends to reinforce negative elements. In the words of Anneli Stranz, we encounter an 'invisible crisis', which relates to working conditions that have a detrimental impact upon care for the elderly. In this vicious circle, care needs are not met, with serious implications for care.

Neoliberal care implies an increasing role of the market, market values and identities within the state and in society. Caring services are outsourced, while some care becomes the responsibility of families and significant others – or even civil society (volunteering). This is what we call 'caring on market terms'. It includes turning care into a product that has to be customer and service orientated, together with the ubiquitous management strategies and, most recently, financialisation – or corporatisation – of care. Corporatisation involves the growing presence of large, for-profit companies, the adoption of corporate practices (cost-cutting, business management models) and a general reconfiguration of care (Farris and Marchetti, 2017: 116) (also see Chapters 3 and 4).

Management and technological fixes are seen as the solutions to the problems in care, yet both Hoppania et al (Chapter 6) and Kovalainen (Chapter 4) in this book argue that it is part of the care crisis because both solutions reduce the complexity of the problems regarding care. The care crisis continues because care is difficult to manage and because the prevailing management strategies conflict with the logics of care. This is also the case regarding the lack of resources, both financial and in terms of the labour force. The latter is an increasing problem, because poor working conditions are causing care workers to want to leave the sector (also see Chapter 5).

What about gender equality and welfare state sustainability?

The beginning of this book asked about the concerns regarding gender equality and welfare state sustainability. When examining the consequences of the care crisis for gender equality, we do not discuss changes in gender equality policies and discourses, but focus on the lived and gendered effects of care policies and neoliberal ideals of care as well as gender equality and social justice in relation to care. The major questions are: What is the status of care work/social reproductive work? What are the possibilities to care for oneself and others? Are societal resources distributed to care sufficient to create a sustainable society? What is the state of the institutions, compromises and contracts[2] that historically have supported gender equality? Do care policies support an equal and just society?

Many of these questions do not have a simple answer, but reveal contradictory developments and the need for further research. An example is the status of paid care work, which on the one hand is highly professionalised and covered by labour market regulation and collective agreements, and on the other hand is subordinated productive work regarding pay and is under pressure from – and rewritten by – market discourses. There is a lack of resources leading to intensified workload, poor working conditions and health problems among care workers. Besides the gender pay gap being rather consistent, an increase in precarious work raises new issues regarding income and independence. A specific concern is the increasing number of migrant workers in social reproductive work with low pay and poor working conditions. Another concern is the increasing pressure on unpaid care work. Finally, it is evident that both the class compromise and care compromise are being challenged, yet not abandoned. The latter is also of importance to the discussion on welfare state sustainability.

In Fraser (2016), a care crisis might develop into a societal crisis if the exploitation of care work (formal as informal) as well as carers (paid as unpaid) leads to a break-down of social reproduction. Is this in the pipeline for the Nordic welfare states? Is a care crisis making the Nordic welfare states less sustainable?

While gender equality is discussed both in the introduction and throughout the book, welfare state sustainability is less developed both as a concept and in the chapters. This is, however, not only a problem in our book: there is no clear and commonly agreed definition of welfare state sustainability; and in general, varied and unclear definitions are commonplace in research on sustainability (Langergaard and Dupret, 2020). Moreover, Schoyen and Hvinden (2017: 317) argue that 'the dominating conceptions of "welfare state sustainability" are rather narrow', because they only consider/exclusively focus upon social outcomes and financial considerations.

In this volume, concerns regarding care work are transversing climate and environmental, economic, and social sustainability; and welfare state sustainability is seen as an overarching concept. We agree with Fraser (2014, 2021) and Langergaard and Dupret (2020) that the three forms are mutually dependent and that sustainability should be discussed as an integrated perspective which concerns deep structures and fundamental values in society.

The Brundtland report, which is one of the first major contributions to the sustainability theme, discusses interlocking crises following human development and demonstrates how 'efforts to guard and maintain human progress, to meet human needs, and to realise ambitions are simply unsustainable – in both rich and poor nations' (World Commission on Environment and Development, 1987: 8). We argue that the care crisis has to be included in the discussion of interlocking crises to be able to understand fully the depth and extent of societal crisis.

The Brundtland report argues that sustainable development includes meeting the basic needs of all, including that the poor get a fair share of the resources, and that the political system should secure democratic participation of all citizens in the making of a sustainable work. However, they emphasize that that 'sustainable development is not a fixed state of harmony, but rather a process' (World Commission on Environment and Development, 1987: 9). In a newer version, sustainability is connected to creating a dignified life for all human beings 'through a combination of economic development, social inclusion, and environmental sustainability' (Hildebrandt, 2016: 15). Moreover, the literature on sustainability points at the importance of structures, institutions, regulations, and social relations in reaching a sustainable world (Dillard et al, 2008; Hildebrandt, 2016; Langergaard and Dupret, 2020; Schoyen and Hvinden, 2017). Following this argument, our conclusion as a whole is a discussion of challenges to the sustainability of the Nordic welfare states. We will, however, highlight a few points here:

- In our book, economic and social sustainability are perspectives closely related to the discussion of class and care compromises. Policy mechanisms and institutional arrangements remain prevalent, yet the care crisis challenges the existing representation of interests and the balancing of power. On the other hand, social justice struggles build solidarity and social cohesion, and show, in reality, how sustainable development is an ongoing process requiring collective action and wise leadership (see also Hildebrandt, 2016). This book shows how individual protest and collective action have highlighted the importance of care, and when successful, have reduced the consequences of, or even hindered or rolled back, existing policies.
- In the original contribution from the World Commission on Environment and Development, distribution was discussed as a matter of class and generation; later, gender was added and as societies in the Global North have become increasingly diverse, matters of distribution regarding race/ethnicity have to be included. The contributions in this book show how the maldistribution of societal resources leads to intensified workload, poor working conditions and health problems. Pay is also unequally distributed between social reproductive work (mainly women's work, mainly public sector) and productive work (mainly men's work in the private sector). Furthermore, an increase in ethnic minority workers in low-paid social reproductive jobs adds to the problem of distribution.
- Do care professionals and care workers lead a dignified life? The discussions show that care professionals and care workers experience disrespect and that care work as such suffers from lack of recognition. In some cases, this occurs to an extent that it affects the health and well-being of the carers.
- Esping-Andersen (2000) discusses how welfare policies do not meet the challenges to welfare state sustainability and even risk enforcing these. We will point at how the two major strategies to solve the care crisis, leadership and technology risk deepening the care crisis.

We have not discussed environmental and climate sustainability, but Schoyen and Hvinden rightly argue that 'climate change and associated politics interact with issues of social policy and welfare state institutions' (2017: 371). They highlight how climate change raises a number of problems regarding social justice and distribution. From the perspective of this book, a particular concern is if the environmental crisis both deepens already existing problems with social injustice *and* creates new problems; this interacts with the care crisis and enforces the pressure on welfare state sustainability.

The Nordic welfare state: a virtuous circle with vicious elements?

This book has identified an uneven and variegated care crisis in the Nordic welfare societies. It could then be argued that the care crisis is less severe than in liberal and continental welfare regimes. But is it at all possible to speak about different levels of a care crisis? One way to approach this is by discussing the care crisis as a continuum with care crisis tendencies at one end (few indicators) and a full care crisis indicating a deep societal crisis threatening welfare state sustainability at the other (containing all indicators of a care crisis). However, this is not a dynamic model and is therefore less suitable for including contradictory developments. It might therefore be more helpful to think of this as a circle.

Joan Tronto (2013) describes a vicious circle in which care is primarily thought about in market terms. Neoliberalism puts competition and profit-making at the centre, resulting in insufficient care and inequalities in care-giving and care-receiving. This book has highlighted several examples of caring on market terms and how they add to the care crisis, as well as the existence of vicious circles within, for example, elder care. But is it possible also to speak about a virtuous circle? If only indicators of a care crisis are included in the discussion, this will not provide the full picture of the state of the care crisis. Other factors also need to be considered: labour market regulations, politics, discourses, institutions and actions, which support care, care workers, gender equality and welfare state sustainability, and mitigate the care crisis. Tronto (2013, 2015) develops the ideal of 'a caring democracy', which is best described as the opposite of caring on market terms. It includes, among other things, solidarity, social justice, responsibility, deliberative commitment and caring institutions *and* making the economy support a 'care-filled life' and not the other way around (Tronto, 2015). All these elements add to a 'virtuous circle'. Likewise, Doellgast et al (2018) contend that we can speak about a virtuous circle which build on inclusive institions, inclusive solidarity and inclusive union and employer strategies, which results in reducing precarious work. In both Tronto's theoretical reflections and Doellgast et al's empirically generated model, many features of the Nordic welfare state and labour market models are included, which indicate that these could form the basis for a virtuous circle.

Following many years of neoliberal politics, the Nordic welfare state has changed. However, this book shows that neither the fundamental values nor the basic institutions have been abandoned. The balance of power in the Nordic class compromise and Nordic care compromise is being challenged, but the platform for solving conflicting interests between capital (employers' organisations) and labour (trade unions) still exists, as do the policy mechanisms and institutions which moderate the contradiction between production and social reproduction. Care services are still accessible, although to varying degrees, and generally free of charge. Care workers are mostly professionals and mainly employed in the public sector, although major differences exist between the Nordic states as to the degree of outsourcing. Care professionals are almost all union members and their work is covered by collective agreements and other forms of labour market regulation. Welfare services are tax-financed, and care politics and the organisation of care are handled by democratic institutions.

In addition, changes are not just happening; they are being fought over, making visible the fact that the Nordic societies are not on a one-way street to a deep crisis. Labour market regulation and institutions give room for social struggles, such as collective bargaining rounds. Workers, their trade unions, citizens and civil society organisations have been able to reduce some of the consequences of the care crisis, while not turning it back. There are also other contradictory elements, such as when gender equality policies and labour market strategies call for men to take part in care work as fathers and workers and for women to participate full-time in the labour market. This is not only reproducing a male norm regarding which labour counts as work and making 'mothering' invisible, as argued in Chapter 3; it also makes 'the other half of humanity' responsible for care and disturbs the gender segregation of work, which is part of the problem in the devaluing of care, as argued in Chapter 8. Another example is how professionalisation is a double-edged sword: both a strategy for valorisation of care work *and* a discourse which tends to undermine care work (see Chapters 8 and 9). Finally, COVID-19 has on the one hand continued the pressure on care professionals, cleaners and informal carers, while on the other hand has simultaneously made visible the necessity of care work to the survival and well-being of societies – relabelling care as 'essential work'. In some cases, this has even let to an awareness of the need to improve the quality of care work, at least temporarily, as Stranz emphasises (see Chapter 5, and also the Postscript).

Does the Nordic context, then, make up a virtuous circle, but with vicious elements? Or is it the opposite way around, a vicious circle with virtuous elements? It is important to remember that the background for talking about a virtuous vis-à-vis vicious circle is the prevalence of neoliberalism and its impact on care work globally. Simultaneously, the contradictions between capital and labour and production and social reproduction are becoming more pronounced, and as concluded in the previous section, the Nordic welfare states are becoming less sustainable. However, as Fraser (2016) shows, Keynesian state strategies can reduce the consequences of this development. The Nordic welfare state model does not comprise a virtuous circle in itself; it may, however, provide the basic elements to moderate the crisis. A salient point, which can be learned from this book, is that any discussion on virtuous vis-à-vis vicious circles *and* any attempt to build a model of a virtuous or vicious circle have to consider that when focus is shifting from regulations, institutions and fundamental values *to* micro processes in everyday life, then the care crisis becomes evident.

The 'caring' states as a critical case

Having reached the end of this book, there is no doubt that we can speak about a care crisis in the Nordic welfare states. This care crisis is occurring in a context where it is most unlikely to appear: that of the 'caring' states. Following Flyvbjerg's (2006) critical case definition, it is therefore plausible to argue that if it is valid here, it applies to all cases; hence, care crisis tendencies are a more widespread phenomenon, relevant to all capitalist (Western) societies. This book points at three important insights about the care crisis, which extend beyond the Nordic setting. Firstly, it highlights the contradictory and complex nature of the care crisis. Secondly, it reveals how management strategies and technological fixes add to the crisis. And finally, it shows how the current professionalisation discourse tends to undermine basic elements of care work. It is also clear from the discussions in this book that even though the fundamental elements of the care crisis are the same across nation states and some features are shared, it is important to place the care crisis within a national context (paying particular attention to the gender and care regimes): the care crisis does not surface in the same way everywhere.

Throughout this chapter, we have discussed the many ways in which the care crisis surfaces in the Nordic welfare states. Here, the focus is on three tendencies. Firstly, informal/unpaid care is under pressure. This might be the case everywhere but in the specific Nordic content, the importance of unpaid care work to society is becoming increasingly invisible while at the same time there is increasing demand for – and attempt to govern – 'someone' to do the work. The COVID-19 crisis has made this dilemma clear as parents were expected to continue working from home while at the same time taking care of their children when day-care institutions and schools were closed. At the same time, the pressure to participate in the labour market is intensifying because of cuts to social security as well as a reinforced political discourse on full-time employment. Another specific variant is the devaluation of mothering and strong emphasis on fathering. Secondly, there is a special version of financialisation in which tax contributions are used for profit-making through outsourcing and privatisation of welfare services. And finally, there is a triple-sided insight that welfare institutions, labour market regulations and influence channels are almost unchanged while at the same time workplace conditions and the logics of care are fundamentally changed. Yet, the very same institutions, regulations and channels of influence provide room for resistance. This renders visible the complexity of the crisis.

Care in the future: three questions for future research and for care activism

This book has provided novel insights on the existence of a complex care crisis in the Nordic welfare regimes. During our discussions, we also noticed research themes that couldn't be looked at within the resources and time available.

Firstly: what do we need to know more about?

This book discusses the Nordic welfare states and societies as one entity and with a focus upon paid care work. It has not sufficiently and systematically taken into consideration the differences in welfare state services, benefits and strategies, as well as the labour market regulation and institutional set-up in the individual Nordic welfare states. This book has barely touched upon differences in gender equality discourses and policies and their relation to care-giving and care-receiving. However, the national context makes a difference to how the care crisis surfaces and its depth, even between Denmark, Finland, Norway and Sweden. Therefore, comparative research is needed on the care crisis in the Nordic context to pinpoint the similarities and differences, but comparative research also needs to be conducted between the Nordic welfare states and other welfare state, labour market and family models, such as, for example, the United States. The discussions in this book indicate that the differences are not only to be found on a national level, but also between different areas of care (for example, hospitals and care for the oldest old), between local governments, and in management strategies and worker influence in workplaces. Earlier research by Dahl (2009) indicates that even within one form of care, care for the elderly within their own homes, there are large differences between municipalities, at least in Denmark.

Another area requiring more analysis – and a different kind of research – is the various ways in which retrenchment of the welfare state and care services can take place. Often there is an analytical focus upon cuts or reduced spending. Although this is sometimes the case, there can be retrenchment even within a stable budget and in the absence of cuts (Dahl 2005). It can take place when care is rearticulated into a 'thinner' ideal of care, stressing self-responsibility of the elderly and coaching them to perform the care themselves (Dahl, 2005, 2012). Retrenchment can also take place when the same number of resources are supposed to cover a larger number of elderly people in need of care, or when care needs to change and intensify, or when new needs emerge. Finally, retrenchment can result when resources within care are directed at standardising and documenting care done instead of doing care.

Finally, welfare state sustainability and the relation to care and social reproduction is an area which needs much more research. This chapter has pointed at elements which need to be included in the discussions on welfare state sustainability, but this needs to be explored in much greater depth.

Secondly: what is a good and just life for care workers, care givers and care receivers?

One element of concern for the quality of care is 'caring for the carer' (Kittay et al, 2005), which is about the conditions under which care workers and care professionals work. Not much is known about how these conditions have – or do not have – an impact upon the care provided and its quality. Theoretically, a positive relation can be assumed between better working conditions in terms of sufficient time for the care to be provided (realistic workload) and an expectation of better care. This book has touched upon this in Chapters 5 and 7, but more research needs to be conducted on this issue. Moreover, increasing 'hiccups' of inadequate care, that is, care scandals (Hoppania and Vaittinen, 2014), need to be explored. Therefore, there is a need to discuss ideals of care, care as a matter of social justice and what determines a good life as a care worker. This is not only a question for (action) research, but also a democratic task, involving the development of deliberative processes which can include the voices of care workers, care-givers, care-receivers, their significant others and institutions. In short, issues of justice need to be related to issues of democracy.

Thirdly, how can this be made possible?

Over the last ten years, an increasing amount of research-based literature has discussed the importance of care/social reproduction not only for feminist research but also for economic theory (Bjørnholt and McKay, 2014; Marcal, 2016; Raworth, 2017) and for social movements (Arruzza et al, 2019; The Care Collective, 2020). Joan Tronto (2013) discusses in her book *Caring Democracies* how it is necessary to move from 'a market-foremost citizen' to a 'caring-foremost citizen'. This interest in care was evident even before the COVID-19 pandemic hit the world. The aim of these contributions is not only to criticise theories and policies and to fight for a higher status of care work; it is to place care and social reproduction at the centre of theory and societies, and to call for another social, economic and political system. Klein (2017) illustrates this in a call for a different society as a solution to the ills of our neoliberal times:

> [W]hen people spoke about the world they wanted, the words *care* and *caretaking* came up again and again ... [T]hat became a frame within which everything seemed to fit: the need to shift from a system based on endless taking—from the earth and from one another—to a culture based on caretaking, the principle that when we take, we also take care and give back. (Klein, 2017: 240–241)

The aim of our book is to improve theorisation, methods and empirical knowledge of the care crisis in the Nordic welfare states. These are issues that are related to the current struggles about care work and social reproduction. Hence, the book may also contribute to a clearer understanding of the background, issues and goals of the social justice struggles.

Notes
1   A governance of details refers to a way of governing that focuses upon codifying, standardising and spelling out the various elements of care by splitting them up into detailed functions.
2   Please see Chapter 3 in this volume for a discussion and definition of class compromise and the counterpart of care compromise. Important is also the understanding of a gender contract, as discussed in Hirdmann (1998).

References
Arruzza, C., Bhattacharya, T. and Fraser, N. (2019) *Feminism for the 99%: A Manifesto*, London and New York: Verso.

Bjørnholt, M. and McKay, A. (eds) (2014) *Counting on Marilyn Waring: New Advances in Feminist Economics*, Bradford: Demeter Press.

The Care Collective (2020) *The Care Manifesto: The Politics of Interdependence*, London and New York: Verso.

Dahl, H.M. (2005) 'A changing ideal of care in Denmark: A different form of retrenchment' in H.M. Dahl and T.R. Eriksen (eds) *Dilemmas of Care in the Nordic Welfare State*, Aldershot: Ashgate, pp 47–61.

Dahl, H.M. (2009) 'New Public Management, care and struggles about recognition', *Critical Social Policy*, 29(4): 634–654.

Dahl, H.M. (2012) 'Neo-liberalism meets the Nordic welfare state: Gaps and silences', *NORA – Nordic Journal of Feminist and Gender Research*, 20(4): 283–238.

Dillard, J., Dujon, V. and King, M.C. (eds) (2008) *Understanding the Social Dimension of Sustainability*, London and New York: Routledge.

Doellgast, V., Lillie, N. and Pulignano, V. (2018) *Reconstructing Solidarity: Labour Unions, Precarious Work, and the Politics of Institutional Change in Europe*, Oxford: Oxford University Press.

Esping-Andersen, G. (2000) 'The sustainability of welfare states into the twenty-first century', *International Journal of Health Services*, 30(1): 1–12

Farris, S.R. and Marchetti, S. (2017) 'From the commodification to the corporatization of care: European perspectives and debates', *Social Politics*, 24(2): 109–131.

Flyvbjerg, B. (2006) 'Five misunderstandings about case study research', *Qualitative Inquiry*, 12(2): 219–245.

Fraser, N. (2014) 'Behind Marx's hidden abode. For an expanded conception of capitalism', *New Left Review*, 86(March/April): 55–72.

Fraser, N. (2016) 'Contradictions of capital and care', *New Left Review*, 100(July/August): 99–117.

Fraser, N. (2021) 'Climates of capital. For a trans-environmental eco-socialism', *New Left Review*, 127(Jan/Feb): 94–127.

Hildebrandt, S. (ed) (2016) *Bæredygtig global udvikling. FN's 17 verdensmål i et dansk perspektiv*, København: Jurist- og Økonomforbundets Forlag

Hirdmann, Y. (1998) 'State policy and gender contracts: The Swedish experience' in E. Drew, R. Emerek and E. Mahon (eds) *Women, Work and the Family in Europe*, London and New York: Routledge, pp 36–46.

Hochschild, A.R. (1995) 'The politics of culture: Traditional, cold modern, post modern and warm modern ideals of care', *Social Politics: International Studies in Gender, State, and Society*, 2(3): 331–346.

Hoppania, H.-K. and Vaittinen, T. (2014) 'A household full of bodies? Neo-liberalism, care and "the political"', *Global Society*, 29(2): 70–88.

Kittay, E.F., Jennings, B. and Wasunna, A.A. (2005) 'Dependency, difference and the global ethic of longterm care', *The Journal of Political Philosophy*, 13(4): 443–469.

Klein, N. (2017) *No Is Not Enough: Resisting Trump's Shock Politics and Winning the World We Need*, Chicago: Haymarket Books.

Langergaard, L.L. and Dupret, K. (eds) (2020) *Social bæredygtighed – begreb, felt, kritik*, Frederiksberg: Frydenlund Academic

Lipsky, M. (1980) *Street-Level Bureaucracy: Dilemmas of the Individual in Public Services*, New York: Russell Sage Foundation.

Marcal, K. (2016) *Who Cooked Adam Smith's Dinner? A Story About Women and Economics*, London: Portobello Books

Phillips, S.S. (1994) 'Introduction' in S.S. Phillips and P. Benner (eds) *The Crisis of Care: Affirming and Restoring Caring Practices in the Helping Professions*, Washington, DC: Georgetown University Press, pp 1–15.

Raworth, K. (2017) *Doughnut Economics: Seven Ways to Think Like a 21st-Century Economist*, London: Random House Business Books.

Schoyen, M.A. and Hvinden, B. (2017) 'Climate change as a challenge for European welfare states' in P. Kennett and N. Lendvai–Bainton (eds) *Handbook of European Social Policy*, Cheltenham: Edward Elgar, pp 371–385.

Tronto, J. (2013) *Caring Democracy: Markets, Equality, and Justice*, New York and London: New York University Press.

Tronto, J. (2015) *Who Cares?*, Ithaca: Cornell University Press.

Willliams, F. (2001) 'In and beyond New Labour: Towards a new political ethics of care', *Critical Social Policy*, 21(4): 467–493.

11

Postscript: A care crisis in the time of COVID-19

Laura Horn, Carsten Juul Jensen and Birgitte Ljunggren

Care research does not take place in a vacuum, especially in the context of a global pandemic that has magnified the care crisis dynamics discussed in this book. Perhaps the COVID-19 crisis will actually give impetus to a more enduring, transformative restructuring of care and justice. And yet there is only limited room to reflect on these developments in the format of academic book chapters written mainly in the pre-COVID-19 period. How then can we make sure to position this book in its time, so that you, the reader engaging with our discussions, get a sense of the unsettling, disruptive context in which it has been finalised?

This postscript brings together a range of vignettes by some of the book's contributors on dimensions of COVID-19-related developments in their respective context. Taking the care crisis concept as reference point, each vignette describes a concrete moment, development or process that offers reflections on the discussions in the book within the COVID-19 context. Carsten Juul Jensen provides a glimpse from the perspective of a practitioner of care. Birgitte Ljunggren highlights the ambiguities of the impact of policy reactions to COVID-19, where unintended consequences have indeed shown what early childhood care could look like if there was sufficient political will. Carsten Juul Jensen's poetic rendering of an interview with a nurse volunteering for the COVID-19 unit conveys a feeling of how mundane and at the same time existential hospital care is, on so many levels. Finally, in a reflection on what it means to write and edit a book on the care crisis, Laura Horn highlights the disruptive context of academic work in the time of COVID-19.

When attentive compassionate care becomes dangerous

Carsten Juul Jensen

The man in the bed is skinny and marked by advanced Kaposi's sarcoma. He only has a few days left to live. Arms, head and neck on the man in the bed are covered by the large brown stains that are characteristic of this type of cancer. Sometimes he cries. No one knows if it's of pain or sorrow. Two women are silently doing their job in the naked room where the windows are never opened and where the only exit is a sluice room into the yard. It's an older nurse and a younger nurse. The older nurse has worked at Roslagstulls infektionssjukhus for many years. The younger just started. They've been helping each other change the bandage on one of the man's bedsores and the younger nurse has temporarily taken her dirty gloves off, maybe to adjust a sheet. Suddenly she leans in over the young man in the bed and wipes off a tear with the back of her hand. She does it without thinking in a sudden bout of empathy and compassion. 'I hope you're going to properly sanitise your hands!' They've just stepped out of the sluice room – all the wards are isolated with two doors that can never be open at the same time – and are standing in the yard outside the barracks between two isolation wards. The older can't contain herself but hisses at the younger. 'Yes, if you're going to wipe away tears you need to use gloves'.[1]

The COVID-19 situation reminds me of the time when HIV/AIDS became a worldwide problem, as Jonas Gardell illustrates in this quote. The first nurses who worked in hospitals with people with HIV/AIDS wore protective equipment to protect all the parts of their bodies against infection when they had contact with patients. The extent of the risk of infection was unknown at the beginning of the HIV/AIDS pandemic and the care staff worked according to the same guidelines that are used now for patients that have COVID-19.

On TV, I saw images of people who died from COVID-19 being driven away in trucks. I struggled with the thought that people had to die alone when their relatives were not allowed to visit them in the hospital, as was happening at the time. I put the critical researcher in nursing on the shelf and signed up for the emergency nursing staff so I could at least assist by holding the hands of dying people.

On the way to the closest hospital to participate in an introduction for this emergency job, I passed a white tent in front of the hospital where guards were ready to direct the people there to get tested for COVID-19. The introduction was efficient and application oriented with information about COVID-19, exercises in putting on protective equipment (gloves, lab coat, mask and face shield) and an introduction to the electronic system for documentation.

On my way home, I felt ready to get to work and I felt pride in my body to be a part of a community of health-care professionals that out of solidarity want to work for the patients and break the COVID-19 infection in the white tent and among the emergency nursing staff.

Later I showed up for the first of two planned training shifts in a geriatric unit where six members of staff were away due to illness. I was happy because it has always been a pleasure for me to work with older patients that have lived long and interesting lives, who are not as careful with norms and rules anymore.

It turned out that the six people who were away due to illness had COVID-19. I was a bit worried because my boss had said I was still expected to go through with the online-based teaching and my partner wasn't exactly pleased that I'd signed up for the emergency care staff. My partner and I had fought intensely because I thought he was selfish, but in reality he was worried that he would get infected. He has asthma and would not be able to work if he got COVID-19.

I had to follow two nursing aides that stood shoulder to shoulder by the computer while they planned the tasks of the day. In the breakroom they helped themselves to bread and candy with bare hands.

I had watched a YouTube video about putting on protective equipment according to the right procedure the night before to protect myself, my partner, colleagues and patients. But it turned out not to be necessary – the nursing staff stood close to the patients without protective equipment when they were serving food, helping with baths or in the bathroom. At first, it shocked me: "But don't you put on protective equipment?" I asked. "You can just put on one of those plastic aprons and gloves, if you'd like," was the response.

At first, I decided not to tell my partner.

A guideline had been formulated for the people who worked in the actual COVID-19 sections but apparently there was no guideline for the units that had patients who did not have COVID-19.

I biked home past the white tent. The guards sat on a couple of chairs and I signed out of the emergency care staff list.

It looks nice on the surface with tents, perfect introduction programmes for the emergency nursing staff and good guidelines for the 'real' COVID-19 units. It is not quite as nice behind the scenes, such as in a geriatric unit where the rising number of complexly and acutely ill older patients are admitted. The nursing staff did everything in their power to create a functional everyday environment while they offered the lovely sick elderly patients compassionate, considerate care in textbook fashion. It has become dangerous to wipe tears away without gloves, lab coat, mask and face shield but I could not live with the idea that it was up to my own personal discretion to make the decision to wear protective equipment *if I wanted to*.

192

A few weeks later, the geriatric unit was closed for a while – there were too few nursing staff to care for the older patients – rumour has it they infected each other.

The COVID-19 pandemic: cure for the care crisis in Norwegian early childhood education and care?

Birgitte Ljunggren

24 August 2020, 10.00 am: I find myself behind a disinfected, big meeting table in a bright, modern meeting room at a large conference hotel in Trondheim. I wait for my student group, which I am going to follow for one and a half years as a group moderator and process guide. They are six early childhood centre (ECC) directors studying leadership in a course I teach. Outside, the sun shines; inside, I am excited. It is our first meeting. Due to COVID-19 restrictions, we have moved the first assembly to a conference hotel. There is not enough space at the campus. The teacher team decided that a good way to start such a group session could be to let everybody in the group come up with a situation report, particularly as we all find ourselves in a pandemic. We assumed it must have challenged these leaders, with the strict regulations and lockdown of public life in Norway. This, after all, had left early childhood education centre (ECEC) in a mode of crisis. Firstly, with the lockdown itself, and then later with shorter opening hours, strictly defined cohorts of children together with a fixed team of staff.

24 August 2020, 10.15 am

Birgitte:	So then, let's start with you. How has the spring been for you and your early childhood centre?
Let's call him Al:	This has been the best spring ever, pedagogically and for really caring! Finally, we saw the contours of the ECEC we dream of! Can you imagine – shorter opening hours and fixed and stable staff according to a staffing norm that was good for the children! There has never been so much staff present at work together with the children. There have never been so many happy and content children! They got shorter hours at the centre because of the short opening hours, they got more time together with their parents and we could offer them pedagogical content all day. Of course, the restrictions posed some practical challenges, but everybody wanted to help in solving them.

The local newspaper Adresseavisen *on 11 June 2020*

The municipal executive for education Camilla Trud Nereid would like to suggest a pilot project with reduced ECC opening hours to the Trondheim City Council because of the positive experiences in ECEC during COVID-19. She argues that it has given the children a better pedagogical service because there are more staff present in the shorter opening hours. This is stated in an additional note to her case document file sent to the municipal executive board: 'Based on our experiences with running ECEC during the corona period, the municipal executive for education will assess whether opening hours in the municipal ECCs should be changed to better the staff density. The municipal executive for education will return with a political case about this.' In the same newspaper article, she is supported by an ECEC director. Nereid confirms that she attempts to do this in her role as bureaucrat before the summer holiday starts. The journalist has also interviewed parents:

> 'My working time is from 08.00–15.30 and then I will have to get from work to the ECC to pick up the children. My husband works at the hospital, normally to 16.30. So if reduced opening hours will become normal, I do not know who will take care of our children,' a mother says.

The local newspaper Adresseavisen *on 16 June 2020*

Heading: Cancels shorter ECC opening hours

The Trondheim mayor Rita Ottervik (Social Democrat) closes the discussion about reduced opening hours in the ECCs of Trondheim, before the municipal administration has even presented its case. 'This is not a debate I want to expose people to', she says.

In the same newspaper article, the representative for the Norwegian Confederation of Enterprise (NHO) is cited with the request that this idea must be 'killed before it is born'.

Nurse Karen works in the COVID-19 unit in a hospital

Carsten Juul Jensen

A poetic representation inspired by critical feminist methods to provide an interview with Nurse Karen who voluntarily accepted work at a unit for COVID-19 patients. The interview was conducted in spring 2020 in a former Department of Medical Gastroenterology.

Welcome
we showed up for our first shift
at a department that was totally deserted
like a bomb
everyone had run from
no:
chairs, tables, beds, duvets, coffee cups or people
the introduction poster for the bedpan washer had been removed
many of the nursing staff stand shoulder to shoulder by
the computer

A menopausal lady
hot flashes
hands sanitised for 30 seconds

blue lab coat tied around the waist and neck
blue mask tied well on the back and squeezed tightly around
the nose

face shield on
gloves preferably long on
ready to care for patients
Mrs Jensen
needs help with:
bed bath
getting dressed
wound care
eating
45 minutes
blue lab coat untied
hands sanitised for 30 seconds
gloves off
hands sanitised for 30 seconds
blue lab coat stripped off
hands sanitised for 30 seconds
mask off
hands sanitised for 30 seconds
face shield off
hands sanitised for 30 seconds

make sure to only touch the clean parts, the parts that have not
been in contact with patients

the menopausal lady is soaked as if she has run a half marathon
the lady needs to go to the changing room in the basement to
change her uniform

did I sanitise my hands when I moved the gloves from the
wrong bin?

Patients
Woman of 45 years is discharged
falls in her home
can't breathe
readmitted

No one will die alone on my shifts
sitting in a lab coat, mask, face shield and gloves
holding hands
can the dying lady feel empathy behind my mask
in the visible part of my body – my eyes

The lady with dementia
who is already confused about where she is
thinks she has landed on an untouched planet
among people in blue with masks and face shields
who are you?

Remember that the doorknob is unclean – friend: sanitise
your hands

COVID-19
The hygiene nurse knows all the hygiene rules
not afraid of infection
heavy breath

Covid-19 negative

training for the run across the Storebælt bridge for a half marathon
must give up after 12 km
can't anymore

Covid-19 positive

Sick

fever with breathing difficulties in a big house isolated from family

Healthy
back in the Ambulatory Endoscopy Clinic
Covid-19 unit closed
tired

heavy breath
Hope to be ready for running a 4k in the future

I hope this email finds you well

Laura Horn

And then COVID-19 came. Within the Nordic Care Crisis research network (NCCN), we had been working on this book about the care crisis in the Nordic countries for a while, having organised several workshops and a PhD event over the last few years. Care researchers themselves are subject to the very fact that as academic workers we are humans, not machines. Babies were born, relatives died, bodies fell ill, bodies recovered. Colleagues joined the group, others left the group, as the academic ebb and flow led them. We had planned to finalise the book in late spring 2020, flanked by a big concluding conference in which core findings could be discussed with care practitioners and relevant policy-makers.

In Denmark, where the three editors of this book are based, things happened quickly, in those first weeks in March when people realised that the mysterious virus 'from China' was no longer far away, but rather a serious, global health threat. Watching military vehicles driving bodies out of Bergamo in Italy. Emotional responses trying to cope with fear, anxiety. The lockdown came fast and sweeping, in Denmark, Norway and Finland. In Sweden, the government looked a different approach. People in the Nordic countries looks to their Swedish neighbours, some with jealousy, many incredulously. Uncertainty about how the virus would affect all of us, hospitals, nursing homes. COVID-19 exposed faultlines in care and social reproduction in and across the Nordics that had been hidden from view before. As care researchers, many of the contributors of this book had been writing and ringing alarms about these for a long time. The invocation of solidarity, of *samfundssind* (community spirit, in Danish), points towards possibilities for alternative care practices on the horizon. Would COVID-19 become the vindication of care researchers, when the faint echoes of clapping for nurses had subsided?

The pandemic hit some of us hard. Care responsibilities, existing preconditions making bodies even more vulnerable, uncertainties for research plans, heavy teaching schedules that had to be kept, COVID-19 or not.

Universities were not a top priority for policy-makers, not even a mid-range concern. Our students often felt adrift; lecturers were expected to master the digital turn with some technical help but no compensation of time. In teaching, much time went to simply checking in on students when faced with an online group. Show your face, say hello to my cat, let's help each other understand that we're still a community, even if only through virtual communication. Care practices in teaching matter, too.

Maintaining an editorial voice in a pandemic can be difficult and wearisome: 'Look, we really need you to send us your draft, so that we can send you comments so that there is half a chance you can get the final version to us in time.' How many times can you preface such urgent editorial emails with 'I hope this email finds you well, in these strange times' when what you really want to write is 'No, I'm not fine either'? Academia is not a pony club. COVID-19 is not a cold.

The care practitioners and colleagues we had invited to join us for the conference, one after the other, informed us that they could not participate; it wasn't safe to travel and anyway they were needed where they were. We decided to postpone, negotiating with the funders. So many online events, so much Zoom in our lives in these first months of COVID-19! We wanted to present our work, our discussions about the care crisis, to actual people in an actual room, to use our bodies to talk about bodies, to celebrate that a project we'd all been working on for so long had finally come to fruition and conclusion. Things will be better, more stable in the autumn; if you say it often enough, you might believe it yourself. We found a date, sent out invitations, received registrations. Then the second wave came. In the end, we moved the event online after all. Even if registration numbers were lower, our discussions about the care crisis showed how urgent these themes are, more than ever in the COVID-19 context.

The last hectic weeks of finalising the book manuscript are now over, and what you're holding in your hands has become both more *and* less than what we had planned and hoped, many years ago when sending off the funding application. Less, as there is so much more research to be done! The contributions to this book are of high quality and each address important issues. But during our discussions it has become clear that we have barely managed to scratch the surface of making sense of the care crisis in the Nordic countries and beyond. So we call on you, dear reader, to continue with systematic studies of the restructuring and transformation of care and social reproduction. At the same time, the book is much more than we envisaged. We can only speculate about what the situation will be at the time of actual publication for this book. What has become clear, however, is that COVID-19 has shown that it is in fact possible to prioritise care, and to provide alternative ways of caring – if there is political will. It is our hope that it will not take another pandemic to centre care and social reproduction in socially just and sustainable societies.

Note

1   Translated from Danish. Gardell, J. (2013) *Tør aldrig tårer bort uden handsker. 1. Kærlighed* (Copenhagen: Tiderne Skifter), pp 5–7.

Index

References to tables appear in **bold** type. References to endnotes show
both the page number and the note number (34n6).

A

Adam, B. 160, 161, 162, 165
ageing-in-place, focus on 83–84
apps
  health 67, 69
  mobile surveillance 70
Arruzza, C. 4, 7, 9, 43, 186
autonomy of care workers 7, 51, 110–111,
  148–149, 150, 153
  see also logic of self-governance

B

Baagøe Nielsen, S. 134, 141, 142, 144,
  146, 148, 149, 150, 152, 153, 154
Bacchi, C. 1, 4, 9, 10, 21, 22, 23, 28,
  30, 34n4
Bhattacharya, T. 6, 9, 40, 43
Bjørnholt, M. 2, 5, 43, 44, 49, 50, 52,
  186
boundary struggles 26, 44, 52, 122
  around care work 123–124
  around childcare 143
  around nursing 133, 135
Brundtland report 180

C

capitalism
  production–reproduction
    contradiction 26–27, 39–40, 41–44,
    48, 122–123, 141
  technology investments 73
  see also financialised capitalism
care
  aspects 5
  contested concept 4–5
  vs. social reproduction 5–6
'care compromise', Nordic 45, 53, 54,
  180, 183
care crisis 2–4
  Anglo-American framing of 20–22
  complexity 177–179
  defining 7, 61, 176–177
  global 7, 26–27, 28
  key concepts and rethinking 4–9
  modes present in research 62
  originating in USA 33
care crisis, Fraser's theory of 39–40, 41–44
  and care and social reproduction in
    Nordic welfare societies 44–46

and care crisis tendencies in Nordic
    welfare societies 46–52, 52–54, **53**,
    184–185
  devaluation of care work in
    families 48–50
  dynamics of resistance and change
    50–52, 54
  financialisation of care work 46–48
  misrecognition of mothering 49–50
  core dimensions and indicators 43–44,
    44
care crisis, scientific framing of 20–38
  effects of prevalent care crisis
    representation 30–32
  four types of crisis 31–32
  methodology and positioning 22–24
  representations of care crisis 24–28
  silence and silencing 23–24, 28–30,
    33
'care deficit' 24–25, 26, 27
care models 8, 25–26, 31–32
care plans 84
care squeeze 121–122, 124, 126
  care under pressure 127–128
  between everyday nursing and
    patient-centredness 130–131
  overcoming 133, 134
  understaffing and death of a
    patient 128–130
'caring democracy' 182
'caring states' 3–4, 20
  critical case 4, 13, 41, 86, 184
  see also welfare states, Nordic
childcare *see* early childhood education
    and care (ECEC); early childhood
    education and care (ECEC) in
    Denmark; early childhood education
    and care (ECEC) in Norway
choice, consumer 120, 121, 144
class compromise, Nordic 45, 53, 54, 180,
    181, 183
cleaning industry, Danish 50–51
cold-modern care model 8, 26
collective action 51–52, 181, 183
  'undersköterskeupproret' (the struggle of
    care workers) 94–95
commodification of care 27, 28, 29–30,
    32, 42, 45, 62
competence-raising measures in early
    childhood centres *see* early childhood

education and care (ECEC) in
  Norway, raising quality in ECCs
consumer choice 120, 121, 144
consumers, patients as 69, 120–121
corporate non-responsibility 158,
  172–173
corporatisation of care 47–48, 179
costs of care
  digitalisation of care and 68–69
  projections 64–65
COVID-19 pandemic 60, 183, 190–197
  comparison with HIV/AIDS
    pandemic 191
  compassionate care and risk of infection
    in hospital 190–193
  and early childhood education and
    care 184, 193–194
  highlighting situation in elder care 94
  making necessity of care work
    visible 94, 183
  nursing on a COVID-19 unit
    194–197
  technologies and 67, 68
  and working on this book 197–199

D

Dahl, H.M. 2, 3, 4, 5, 6, 7, 8, 9, 20, 21,
  22, 23, 24, 28, 30, 32, 45, 46, 51, 80,
  81, 82, 85, 101, 104, 105, 106, 123,
  124, 139, 140, 141, 145, 147, 161, 172,
  177, 185, 186
deinstitutionalisation 84
Denmark
  budget cuts and care of elder
    inpatients 125
  cleaning industry 50–51
  education in care work reforms 144
  gender equality 46
  health industry 48
  resistance and struggles over care in
    labour market 50–52
  time-navigating practices in home
    care 161
  see also early childhood education and
    care (ECEC) in Denmark; health
    services in Denmark; nursing
    in Denmark
devaluation
  of care 27, 48 50, 89, 93 94
  of feminine 83, 93
  of mothering 49, 50, 183, 185
division of labour in care work 105
documentation 84, 90, 104, 108
Doellgast, V. 182
dual-breadwinner model 26, 42, 45,
  49, 148
dual-earner-dual-carer model 49, 50,
  177

E

early childhood education and care
  (ECEC) 139, 140
  as care work in crisis 147–152
  OECD recommendations for
    performance measurement 148–149
  status in Nordic countries 143–147,
    152–153
early childhood education and care
  (ECEC) in Denmark 139, 140
  as care work in crisis 147–152
  child-staff ratios and hours spent with
    children 149, **149**, 160
  double-edged sword of
    professionalisation 152–153, 154
  experience of newly graduated
    pedagogue 149–152
  gendered care work 148
  holistic pedagogical approach 150–151
  'learning pedagogy' 146–147
  OECD recommendations for
    performance measurement 148–149
  status of care work 143–147
    organisational and managerial
      reform 145
    social pedagogic tradition and its
      challenges 145–147
early childhood education and care
  (ECEC) in Norway
  background to ECCs 159–160
  concerns over quality 159
  COVID-19 pandemic and 184, 193–194
  education in 160, 162
  expansion of private commercial
    providers 47–48
  at heart of care crisis 158–159
  meagre organisations 159, 167
  percentage of children attending
    ECCs 158
  raising quality in ECCs 162–173
    child-centredness 164–165, 166, 172
    competence-raising measures 163,
      166–167
    daily rhythm 165–166
    filling time gaps with raising of
      competence 169–170
    increasing attention to pedagogy 165
    leaders' temporal orchestration to
      implement competence-raising
      measures 167–169, 172
    methodology 162–164
    motivating staff in
      competence-raising 170–171
    shadowlands of re/production 165,
      166, 167–169, 172, 173
    time in work organisations 160–162
  ratio of staff to children in ECCs 160
  spending on 173

staffing in ECCs 160
tradition of 159–160
early childhood teacher education
 (ECTE) 162
economic crisis 2008 65
economics of care 64–66
 digitalisation of care and 68–69
economisation 60–61, 62
education and training in care work
  84–85, 104, 105, 144, 160, 162
 childcare 143, 149–150, 160, 162
 undermining of nursing 125–126
 unlearning of nursing 131, 133, 135
elder care
 in Danish hospitals 125
 silencing of 29
elder care in Finland 100–119
 crisis of 100–102
 division of labour 105
 funding 103
 improved management seen as solution to
  issues in 100–101, 102–103
 logic of care and limits of detailed
  control 107–109
 logic of care and limits of
  self-governance 109–112
 logic of self-governance 105–107
 managers 104, 105, 106–107, 109–110,
  110–111, 113
 migrant care assistants 105
 professionalism in care 104, 106
 staff turnover 105, 111
 toolbox for managing care
  work 103–107
elder care in Sweden, working
  conditions in
 COVID-19 pandemic and 94
 a gendered issue 80–81, 94
 improving 94–95
 invisibility of care workers 80, 81
 Nordcare study 85–86
 Nordcare study methodology 86–87
 Nordcare study results 87–92
  endangered well-being 91–92
  lack of resources 88–89, 93–94
  physically and mentally demanding
   work 89–91
  relational poverty 91
  unsatisfying employment
   conditions 87–88
  work-life imbalance 88
 shortage of trained staff 84–85
 theoretical approach 82–83
 trends in elder care 83–85
 'undersköterskeupproret' campaign to
  improve 94–95
electronic health records (EHRs) 69
emotions 31, 135
entrepreneurialism 66

Esping-Andersen, G. 3, 20, 45, 140, 181
ethical standards 125–126
ethics of care 60, 61, 108–109, 110
 and moral dimension of care crisis 63–64
 research 62
Evetts, J. 140, 142, 143, 145, 147

F
families
 care deficit in 25
 care in 8, 27, 42, 53, **53**, 177
 devaluation of care work in 48–50
 dual-breadwinner model 26, 42, 45,
  49, 148
 dual-earner-dual-carer model 49,
  50, 177
 ideal of care in 28
 informal elder care 80, 81
 shadowland of work and care in 161
Farris, S.R. 47, 179
fathers 30, 49, 134, 154, 177, 183
financialisation 34n6, 52, 61, 62, 185
 of care work in Nordic welfare state
  context 46–48
 resistance to 52, 54
financialised capitalism 34n6, 49, 53,
  62, 123
 care crisis relating to 21, 27, 28, 39, 40,
  42–43, **44**, 122, 135
Finland *see* elder care in Finland
Fisher, B. 5, 107, 161, 164
Foucault, M. 22, 23, 24
Fraser, N. 2, 6, 7, 8, 9, 21, 22, 24, 26–27,
  28, 32, 34n9, 39, 40, 41–42, 43, 44,
  45, 48, 49, 52, 61, 62, 80, 81, 82, 83,
  87, 88, 95, 122, 123, 124, 140, 141,
  143, 158, 159, 161, 166, 171, 176,
  180, 184
 see also care crisis, Fraser's theory of
future research 185–187

G
gender
 and child care work 148
 and differing experiences of coping with
  performative pressures 133–134
 issue of elder care 80–81, 94
 -segregated labour market 80, 82–83, 93,
  101–102, 183
 specific forms of misrecognition 82,
  83, 93
 stereotypes and robotics 70
 two-dimensional concept of 82–83, **83**
gender equality 8–9, 179–180, 183
 a core dimension of Fraser's care crisis
  theory 44, **44**
 in Nordic countries 44, 45–46, **53**, 54
gender justice 9, 80

perspective on working conditions in
    elder care 87–92, 92–94, 95
two-dimensional model of 82–83, **83**, 87
global care chain 7, 26, 27–28, 33
good care 31, 186
    difficulties in providing 91, 107–108,
        133, 178
    technology within care and
        understandings of 63–64, 71
good-enough care 8, 91, 178
gross domestic product (GDP) 64, 65

H

Hansen, L. 3, 45, 51
health and well-being of carers 108,
    178–179, 181
    burnout 133
    endangered 91–92
    exhaustion 90, 92, 93, 95, 178
    gendered experiences of 133–134
    NQNs' self-blame and sense of
        inadequacy 127–128, 129–130, 131,
        132, 133, 134, 135
    staffing levels impacting 92, 93, 95,
        178–179
    strain of physically and mentally
        demanding work 89–91
health records 66, 69
health services in Denmark 120–138
    accreditation for health-care providers
        (DKKM) 124
    conceptualising crisis of care and drain on
        nursing staff 122–126
    discourses undermining nurses'
        competence 125–126
    elder hospital patients 125
    patient safety friendly hospitals 120–121,
        124–125, 127, 130–131
    study of newly-qualified nurses'
        experiences 127–132
        care under pressure 127–128
        difficulties in conforming with patient-
            centred discourses 131–132, 134
        method and design 126–127
        squeezed between everyday nursing and
            patient-centred care 130–131
        understaffing and death of a
            patient 128–130
    'value for money' and budget
        cuts 124–125
    'We are here for you' slogan 120, 121,
        124, 131, 133
Held, V. 61, 63
Hirvonen, H. 2, 20, 21, 22, 29, 30, 41,
    101, 102, 103, 106, 108, 109, 110
Hochschild, A.R. 7, 8, 9, 24–25, 26, 27,
    31, 176
home care
    in Finland 103, 108, 111

focus on ageing-in-place 83–84
management of tasks 105, 108
in Sweden 84
technologies and 68, 69, 70
time-navigating practices 161
Hoppania, H.-K. 32, 100, 101, 102, 103,
    107, 108, 112, 186
housewifisation 123

I

'illegitimate tasks' 91
informal care *see* unpaid care work
Institutional Ethnography (IE) 122,
    126, 132
Isaksen, L.W. 2, 7, 21, 22, 24, 26, 28, 29, 31

J

Jensen, C.J. 121, 126, 127, 132, 133
justice model, two-dimensional 82–83,
    83, 87
    perspective on working conditions in
        elder care 87–92, 92–94, 95

K

Klein, N. 187
Klikauer, T. 103
Kovalainen, A. 3, 60, 62, 65, 70, 71, 72

L

labour market
    features of women-dominated
        sectors 87–88
    gender-segregated 80, 82–83, 93,
        101–102, 183
    prevalence of women in 148
    regulation 45
    resistance and change in Danish 50–52
lean management principles 161
lifting, heavy 90
Ljunggren, B. 158, 159
Löfven, S. 94
logic of care 101, 112, 113
    applied to care workers and their
        supervisors 111–112
    and limits of detailed control 107–109
    and limits of self-governance 109–112
    temporal 165, 167, 172
logic of details 101, 105, 106, 112
    and logic of care 107–109
logic of self-governance 101, 105–107,
    112–113
    logic of care and limits of 109–112

M

managerialism and care
    management 100–119
    logic of care and limits of detailed
        control 107–109

logic of care and limits of
self-governance 109–112
seeking to improve quality and
efficiency 100–101, 102–103
toolbox 103–107
Marchetti, S. 47, 179
marketisation 42, 46, 60, 65
of health services in Denmark 123, 124,
135–136n1
and management styles 101–102
managerialism and commitment to 120
monitoring of services to
support 84, 152
Martinsen, K. 21, 125, 131, 134, 141
masculinities, changing 30
McKay, A. 2, 43, 186
meagre organisations 159, 161, 167
migration of care workers 7, 26, 27, 61,
85, 105, 180
misrecognition
of care 32, 92, 94
gender-specific forms of 82, **83**, 93
of mothering 49–50, 183
models of care 8, 25–26, 31–32
'modernisation'
discourses undermining nurses'
competence 125–126
of Nordic public services 124–125
professionalisation and 139, 140,
144–145
'monetary care' 65–66
monitoring
of health care services 120–121
to increase ECEC quality 148–149
pressures in childcare work 153
remote health 68, 69
of services to support
marketisation 84, 152
of work performance 67, 70, 72,
104–105, 106, 108
Monrad, M. 159, 173
'moral machines' 72
moral theory, care and 63–64
mothering, misrecognition of 49–50, 183

N

Näre, L. 105
neoliberalising 6–7, 20, 34n1
neoliberalism 3, 6–7, 106
as distinct from financialisation 46–47
and pressure on paid and unpaid care
work 40, 122–123, 135
reframing of care 6–7, 31, 40, 177–178,
179
resistance to changes of 52, 54
New Public Management (NPM) 6, 46,
51, 65, 66, 67, 84, 102–103, 161
performance measurement tools
148–149, 152

reforms in Danish health care 120, 121,
122, 123–124, 134
Niska, M. 106, 109–110
Nordcare study 85–86
methodology 86–87
results from Sweden 87–92
endangered well-being 91–92
lack of resources 88–89, 93–94
physically and mentally demanding
work 89–91
relational poverty 91
unsatisfying employment
conditions 87–88
work-life imbalance 88
Nordic 'care compromise' 45, 53, 54,
180, 183
Nordic class compromise 45, 53, 54, 180,
181, 183
Norway
elder care 85
gender equality 46
paid work and care 49–50
resistance in struggles over care 52
see also early childhood education and
care (ECEC) in Norway
nursing, idealistic understandings of
good 134
nursing in Denmark
care squeeze 121–122, 124, 126
conceptualising crisis of care and drain
on 122–126
discourses undermining educational
competence in 125–126
expert knowledge 126
impacted by discourses of safety
programmes 120–121
knowers 122, 132, 133
study of newly-qualified nurses'
experiences 127–132
care under pressure 127–128
difficulties in conforming with patient-
centred discourses 131–132
squeezed between everyday nursing and
patient-centred care 130–131
understaffing and death of a
patient 128–130
see also health services in Denmark

O

occupational professionalism 142,
145
OECD 2, 64, 66, 142, 143, 146, 147,
148, 160
Olakivi, A. 101, 105, 106, 109–110,
111
orchestration metaphor 162, 168
organisational professionalism 143,
145, 153
outsourcing 51

P

paid care work 40, 43, 45, 80, 85,
  148, 183
  as gendered 54, 80, 83, 93
  problematic representations of
    professional 28
  silencing of professionals in 29–30
  status 179–180
paid work
  prioritised over social
    reproduction 49–50
  women combining care and 3–4, 9, 25,
    40, 42, 44, 161
  women's liberation via 48
parental leave 49
parity in participation 44, 82
part-time work 88, 150
patient-centredness 120–121, 124–125,
  131, 136n2
  difficulties in conforming with discourses
    of 131–132, 134
  squeezed between everyday nursing
    and 130–131
'patient safety friendly hospitals 120, 122,
  124–125, 127, 130–131
pay 87, 93, 181
person-centred care 84, 136n2
personalised health records (PHRS) 69
Phillips, Susan S. 2, 7, 8, 20, 21, 22, 24,
  25, 26, 29, 31, 176
politics of care 61, 66
postmodern care model 8, 25–26,
  31–32
private equity 61, 73n1
private sector
  blurring of public and 60, 65
  care provision in Finland 100, 101
  childcare providers 47–48
privatisation of care work 46, **53**, 62,
  123, 185
professionalisation 3, 125, 139–157
  double-edged sword 152–153, 154
  ECEC as care work in crisis 147–152
  experience of newly graduated
    pedagogue 149–152
  and status of care work with
    children 143–147, 152–153
  strategies and the care crisis 140–143
  theories of 142–143
professionalism 142, 145
  in Finland 104, 106
  holding meetings seen as a lack
    of 170–171
  occupational 142, 145
  organisational 143, 145, 153
public sector
  blurring of private and 60, 65
  care deficit in 24–25

market mechanisms 51–52, 62, 65–66,
  80, 102, 105, 148
paid care work in 40, 45, 54, 80,
  148, 183
privatisation of care work in 46, **53**, 62,
  123, 185

Q

qualifications for care work 141–142
  see also education and training in
    care work
quality control 20, 84, 108, 145
quality of care 47, 89, 100, 178, 186
  difficulties in providing 91, 107–
    108, 112
  numerical data for control of 108
  professionalisation and 143–144
  see also early childhood education and
    care (ECEC) in Norway, raising
    quality in ECCs

R

ratios, staff-child 149, **149**, 160
re-ablement, policy ideals of 32
recognition as social status 82
  see also misrecognition
'regimes of accumulation' 123
relational poverty 91
residential care, elder 88, 94, 103
  reduction in Sweden 84
  scandal in Finland 100
resources
  lack of 88–89, 93–94, 111, 179, 180
  maldistribution of societal 181
  meagre organisations and 159, 161, 167
  preoccupation with numbers 27, 30
responsibility
  corporate non- 158, 172–173
  elder self- 20, 186
  individualisation of 110–111, 173
retrenchment of welfare state 25, 29, 30,
  33, 185–186
rights to receive care 31
robots 70–71, 72
  interfaces with humans 70–71
ruling relations 122, 126–127, 130–131,
  134

S

'self-care' 20, 26, 32
self-governance, logic of *see* logic of
  self-governance
self-management 72–73, 172
shadowlands of work and re/
  production 161, 162, 165, 166,
  167, 173
  leaders' temporal orchestrations
    in 167–169

silencing 23–24, 28–30
single parents 49
Smith, Dorothy 122, 126, 127
social justice 41–44, 181, 182
social reproduction 5–6, 7
  as a 'backward residue' 48
  and care in Nordic welfare states 44–46
  and caring for things, communities and
    the Earth 43
  early childhood care and 47–48, 145,
    146, 158
  prioritising of paid work and erosion
    of 49–50
  –production contradiction 27, 39–40,
    41–44, 48, 122–123, 141
'socioemotional' machines 70
split shifts 88
staff turnover rates 105, 111
staffing levels 89, 93–94, 111
  COVID-19 pandemic and improved
    ECEC 193–194
  in elder care 84–85
  impacting care workers' health and well-
    being 92, 93, 95, 178–179
  negative impacts of understaffing 125,
    128–130
  ratios in childcare 149, **149**, 160
standpoint theory 122
state-managed capitalism 123
Stefansen, K. 30, 50, 52
Stranz, A. 81, 84, 86, 89, 91, 92
stress, workplace 51, 90–91, 93, 95,
    133–134
Suchman, L. 70
supply and demand
  care crisis as an imbalance between
    24–26, 27, 33
  within political economy 26
surveillance mechanisms 67, 68, 69, 70,
    72, 106, 108
  see also monitoring
sustainability, welfare state 180–182
Sweden
  child-staff ratios in childcare 160
  gender equality 46
  home and residential care 84
  see also elder care in Sweden, working
    conditions in
Szebehely, M. 3, 20, 81, 84, 85, 86, 88,
    89, 90, 92, 94, 141, 150

T

Taylorism 104–105, 106, 107–108, 109
techno-political question, care crisis as an
    articulated 66–68
technologies of care 61
  citizen-consumers and use of 69
  innovations in 66

as a 'remedy' to the care crisis 48, 61,
    68–71, 72–73
  and understandings of good care 63–64,
    71
telehealth technologies 68
time in work organisations 160–162
  care and 161–162
  daily rhythm in ECCs 165–166
  filling time gaps 169–170
  leaders' temporal orchestration to
    implement competence-raising
    measures 167–169, 172
  orchestration metaphor 162, 168
time use, conflict over 107–108
Tonkens, E. 16, 81
trade unions 45, 51–52, 143, 183
traditional care model 25
training in care work see education and
    training in care work
Tronto, J. 2, 4, 5, 6, 21, 28, 39, 43, 61, 63,
    82, 107, 161, 164, 182, 186
turnover rates, staff 105, 111
two-earner model 26, 42, 45, 49, 148
two-earner-two-carer model 49, 50, 177

U

'undersköterskeupproret' (the struggle of
    care workers) 94–95
UNESCO 143, 146
universalism of care services 3
unpaid care work 25, 44–45, 72, 177,
    184
  with elderly 80, 81
  in families 8, 27, 42, 48–50, 53, **53**,
    177
  gender as dividing line between paid
    work and 82–83
  lack of status 50, 54
  under pressure 180, 184
  production of economic value based
    on 39–40, 41–43
  women combining paid work and 3–4,
    9, 25, 40, 42, 44, 161

V

'value for money' 124–125, 144
Valvira 100

W

Waerness, K. 39, 80, 107
wages 87, 93, 181
warm-modern care model 26
Weber, J. 70
welfare state sustainability 180–182
welfare states, Nordic
  care crisis dynamics **53**, 177
  care crisis tendencies 46–52, 52–54,
    184–185

devaluation of care work in
  families 48–50
financialisation of care work 46–48
misrecognition of mothering 49–50
resistance to change 50–52, 183
as 'caring states' 3–4, 20
as feminist nirvanas 3–4
modes present in research 62
private sector economic and managerial
  practices 65–66
social reproduction and care 44–46
a virtuous vs. a vicious circle 182–184
women-friendly 3, 8–9, 10, 20, 40–41,
  44–46, 80
'What's the problem represented to be'
  (WPR) 21, 23
Williams, F. 2, 8, 22, 24, 26, 27, 28, 61
Witz, A. 139, 140, 142, 145, 148
work-life imbalance 88
working conditions 178, 180, 186
  and budget cuts in Danish hospitals 125,
    127–132

in COVID-19 pandemic 190–193,
  194–197
deterioration in ECECs 149, **149**,
  153, 160
experience of newly graduated
  pedagogue in ECEC 149–152
monitoring of performance 67, 70, 72,
  104–105, 106, 108
outsourcing and 51
'taskified' 70
time use 107–108
vicious circle of problems of 178–179
see also elder care in Sweden, working
  conditions in
working hours 88, 150
World Commission on Environment and
  Development 180, 181

Z

Zechner, M. 107

Printed and bound by CPI Group (UK) Ltd, Croydon, CR0 4YY

27/10/2024

14580557-0003